HISTAMINE INTOLERANCE COOKBOOK

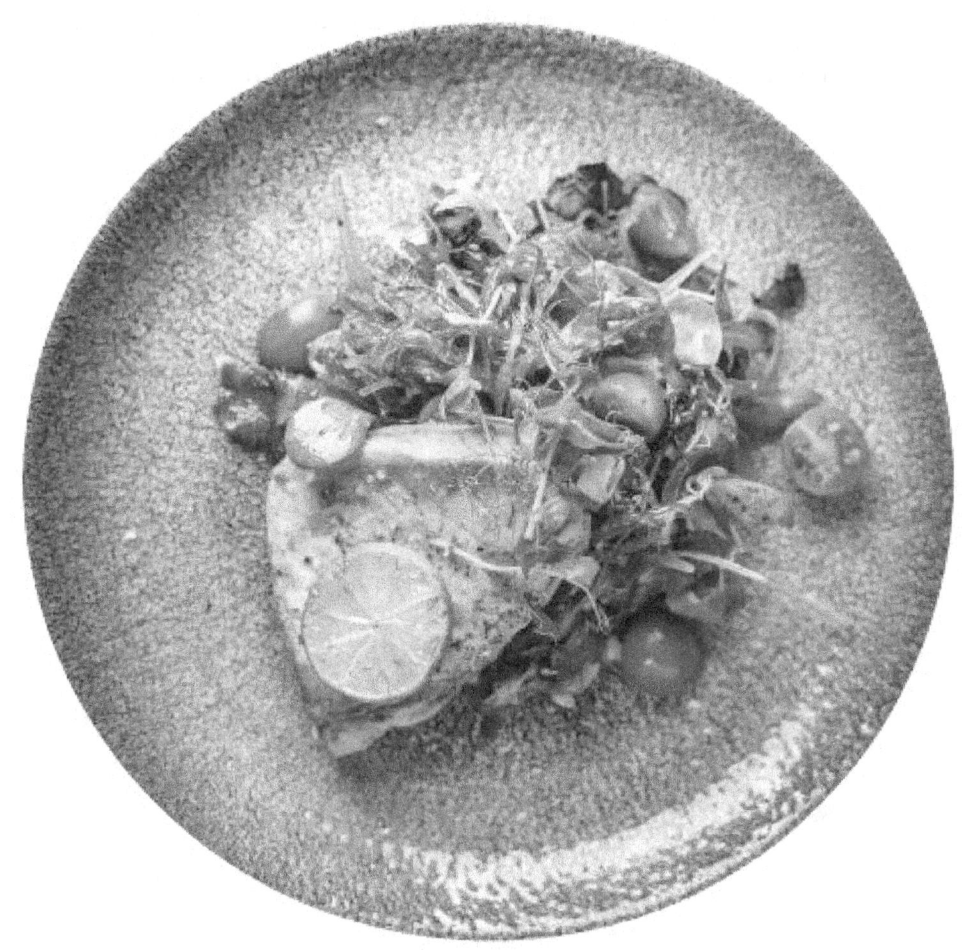

Delicious recipes for Low-histamine diet

Carmen J. Johnson

Copyright © 2024 by Carmen J. Johnson

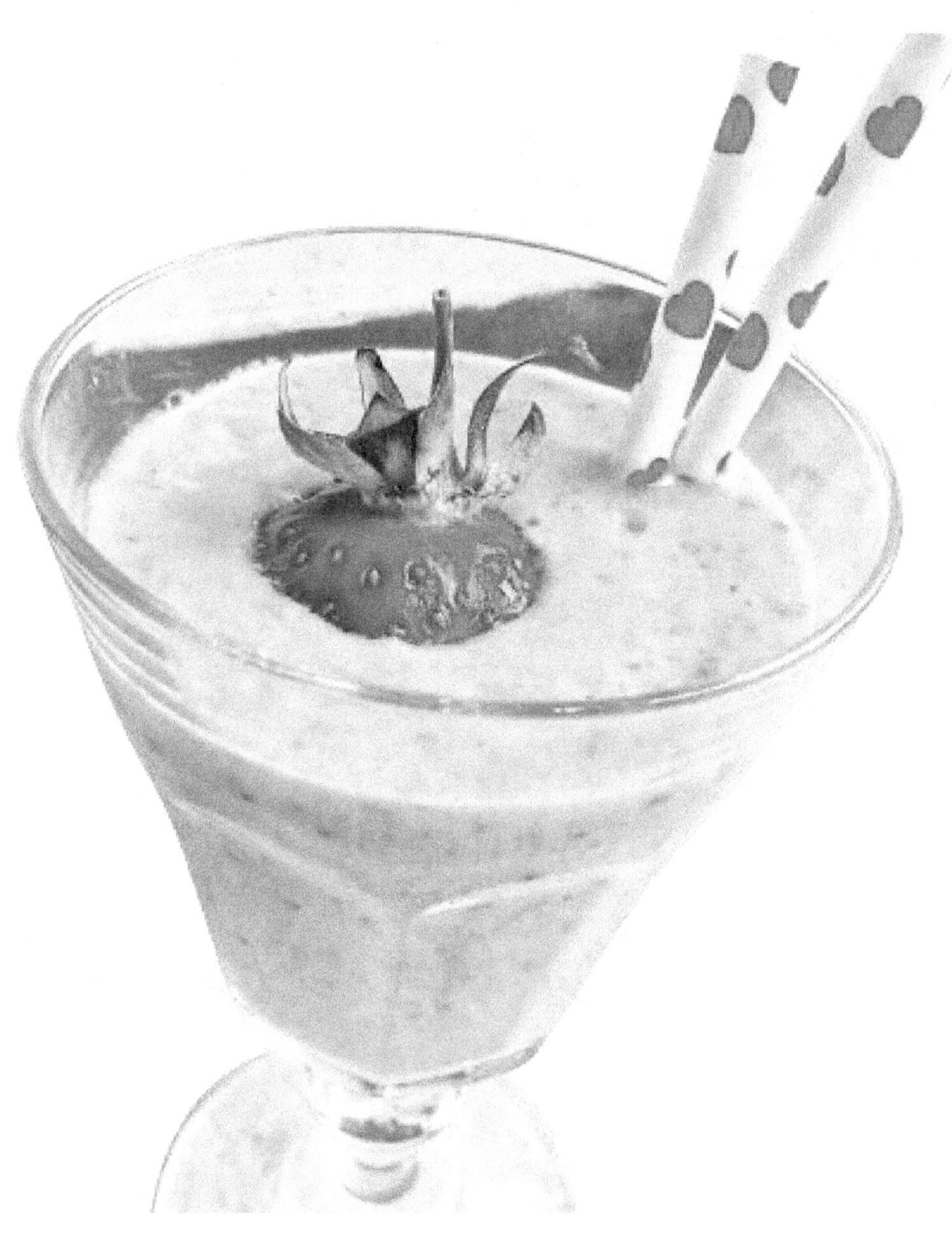

TABLE OF CONTENTS

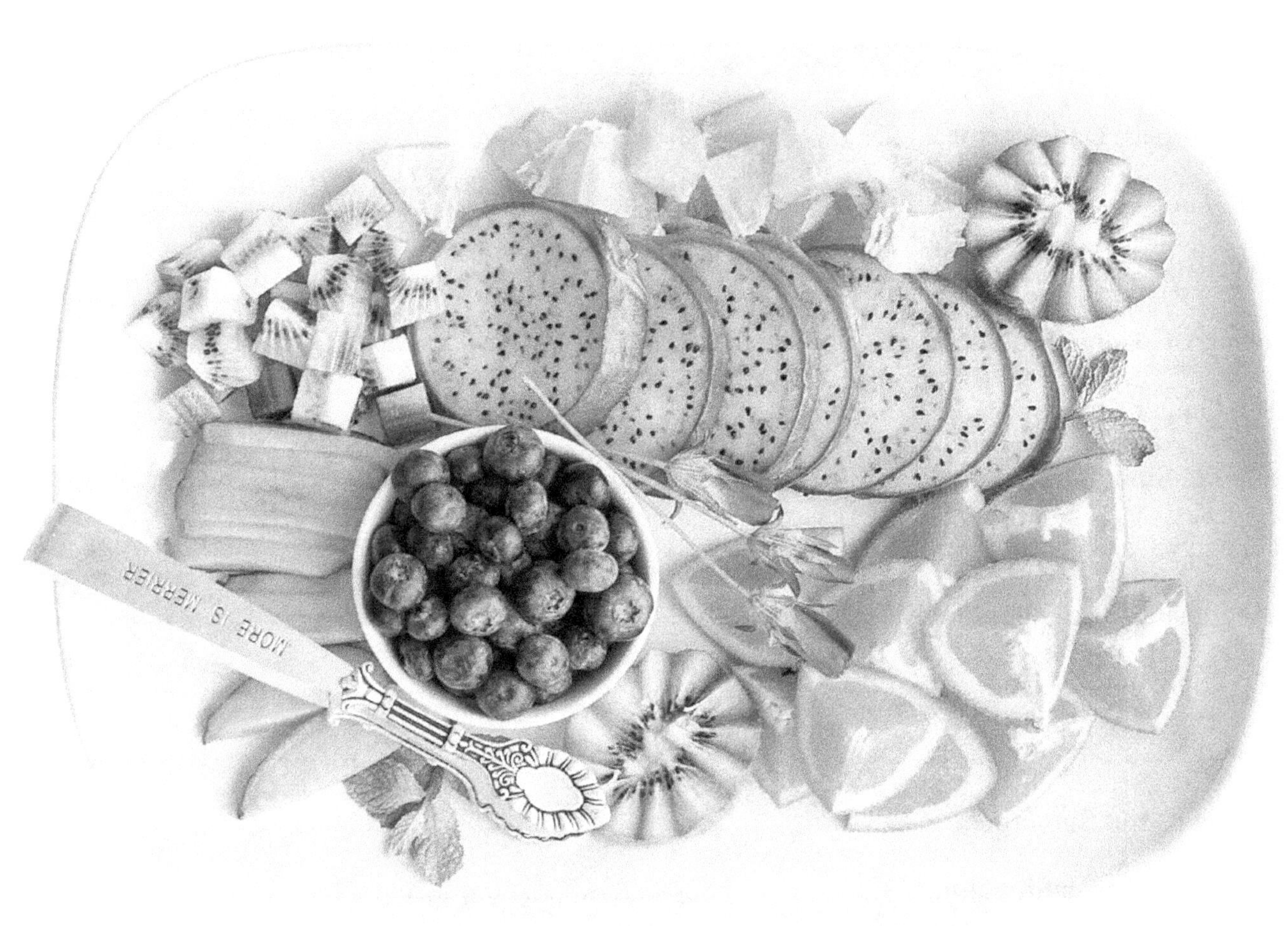

MORE IS MERRIER

INTRODUCTION

Assume you're preparing a wonderful dish, excited about your culinary journey. But instead of the anticipated joy, your body throws a wrench in the works. Headaches throb behind your eyelids, your stomach churns in defiance, and a wave of exhaustion sweeps over you. You're frustrated and perplexed, wondering, "What on Earth just happened?" This, my friends, was my introduction to the mysterious world of histamine intolerance.

For years, I was an avid chef, and my kitchen was a playground of flavors and sensations. However, seemingly benign foods would set off a series of unpleasant sensations. Aged cheese, a dash of fermented tomato sauce, and even a glass of red wine have become culinary culprits. Discouraged and perplexed, I set out on a journey to solve the secret of these emotions.

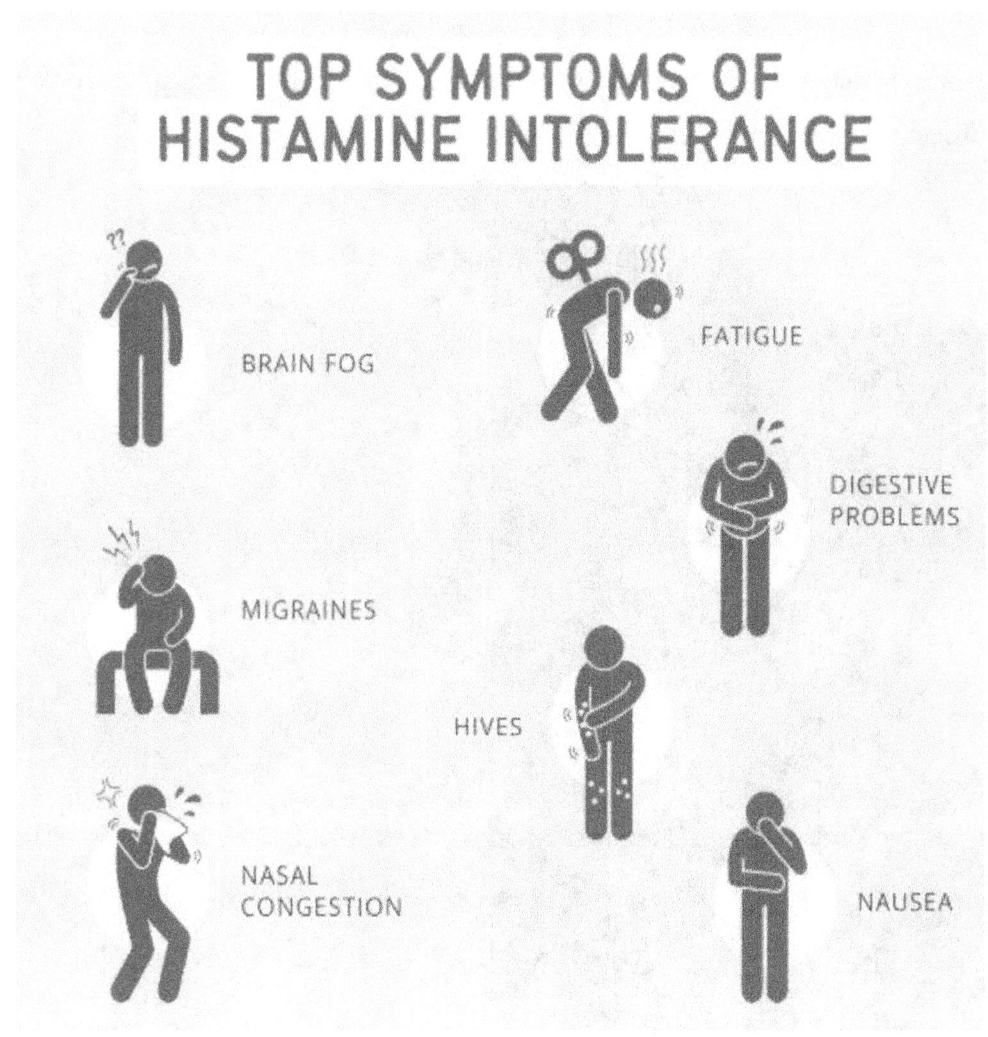

The trek was not easy. Countless online searches and complicated medical terminology left me feeling more overwhelmed than informed. But, gradually, a picture began to develop. I learnt about histamine, a potent molecule in our systems that, when out of balance, may have serious consequences for our health. My body, it found out, was not digesting histamine adequately, making me susceptible to its effects.

But here's some good news: information is powerful.

This knowledge sparked a spark inside me. If I couldn't modify how my body responded to histamine, I could surely adjust my approach to eating. I could see food as an ally rather than a battleground. A voyage of discovery began, in which healthy, low-histamine cooking became the key to recovering my health and reigniting my love of food.

This book commemorates the adventure. It's the result of innumerable culinary experiments, a celebration of great flavors that don't elicit unpleasant emotions, and a guide for those experiencing similar issues.

Instead of a list of constraints, you'll find a universe full of exciting options. We'll look at the theory underlying histamine intolerance, but more importantly, we'll focus on the practical: making tasty, healthy meals that will calm your body and spirit. Whether you're a seasoned chef or a complete novice, join me as we explore the wonderful, flavor-packed world of low-histamine cuisine.

Together, we'll show that controlling histamine intolerance does not have to mean giving up flavor or enjoyment. Let us go on this culinary journey, one delicious low-histamine recipe at a time.

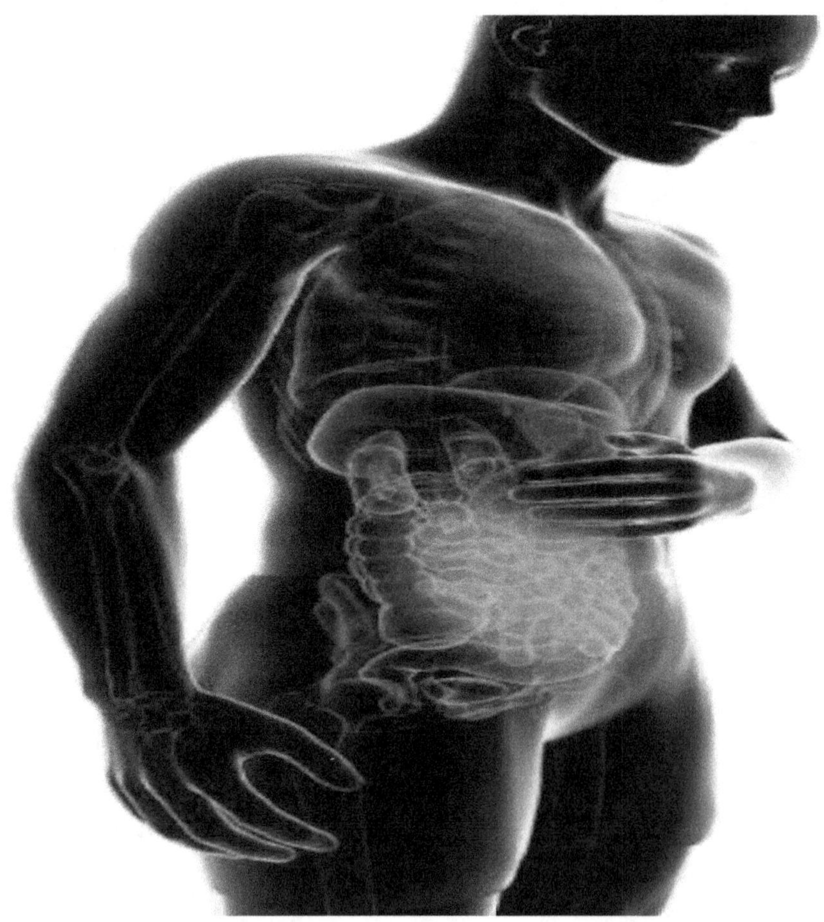

UNDERSTANDING HISTAMINE INTOLERANCE

Understanding histamine and its impact on health

Histamine is a biogenic amine that plays a vital role in the body's immune response, acting as both a neurotransmitter and a local immune system mediator. It is synthesized from the amino acid histidine by the enzyme histidine decarboxylase. Histamine is stored primarily in mast cells and basophils, which are types of white blood cells, and is released in response to injury, allergic reactions, and immune responses.

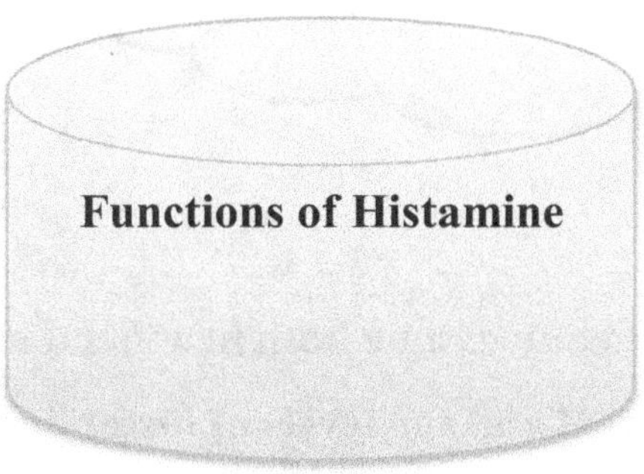

Histamine has several key functions in the body

Immune Response: Histamine is crucial in the body's defense mechanisms. When the body detects an allergen or pathogen, histamine is released from mast cells and basophils, leading to an increase in the permeability of blood vessels. This allows white blood cells and other proteins to move quickly to the site of infection or injury.

Gastric Acid Secretion: In the stomach, histamine stimulates the secretion of gastric acid by binding to H2 receptors on the parietal cells of the stomach lining. Food digestion requires the presence of this acid.

Neurotransmission: As a neurotransmitter, histamine is involved in the regulation of various functions in the brain, including the sleep-wake cycle, appetite control, and cognitive functions.

Inflammatory Response: Histamine contributes to the inflammatory response by causing vasodilation and increasing vascular permeability. This leads to symptoms such as redness, swelling, and heat at the site of an injury or infection.

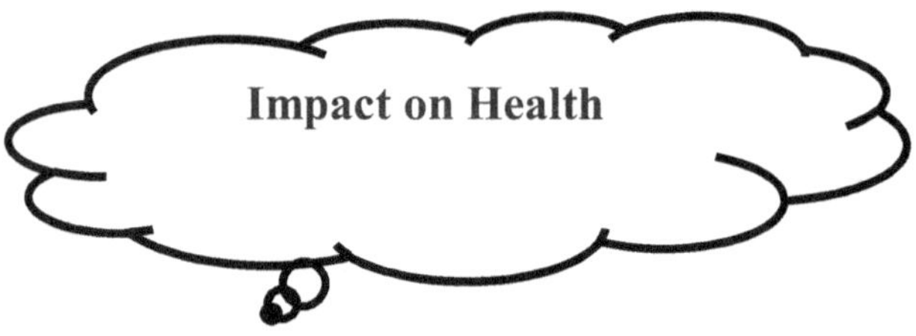

The effects of histamine on health can be both beneficial and detrimental, depending on the context and the levels of histamine present.

Allergic Reactions: Histamine is a major player in allergic reactions. When an allergen enters the body, the immune system overreacts, causing a release of histamine. This leads to symptoms such as itching, hives, runny nose, and watery eyes. In severe cases, it can cause anaphylaxis, a life-threatening condition characterized by difficulty breathing, a drop in blood pressure, and loss of consciousness.

Histamine Intolerance: Some individuals have a condition known as histamine intolerance, where they cannot break down histamine properly due to a deficiency in the enzyme diamine oxidase (DAO). This can lead to symptoms such as headaches, digestive issues, skin problems, and respiratory symptoms. Managing histamine intolerance often involves dietary changes to avoid histamine-rich foods like aged cheeses, smoked meats, and certain alcoholic beverages.

<u>**Chronic Inflammation:**</u> Excessive histamine release can contribute to chronic inflammatory conditions. Conditions like mast cell activation syndrome (MCAS) involve the inappropriate release of histamine and other inflammatory mediators from mast cells, leading to symptoms that can affect multiple organ systems.

<u>**Gastrointestinal Disorders:**</u> Histamine plays a role in various gastrointestinal disorders. Excessive histamine release in the stomach can contribute to peptic ulcers and gastroesophageal reflux disease (GERD) by increasing gastric acid secretion. Conversely, histamine blockers, such as H2 receptor antagonists, are used to treat these conditions by reducing acid production.

<u>**Neurological Effects:**</u> In the brain, abnormal histamine levels have been associated with several neurological and psychiatric conditions. For example, low histamine levels are linked to narcolepsy, a sleep disorder characterized by excessive daytime sleepiness. On the other hand, elevated histamine levels have been implicated in conditions such as schizophrenia and multiple sclerosis.

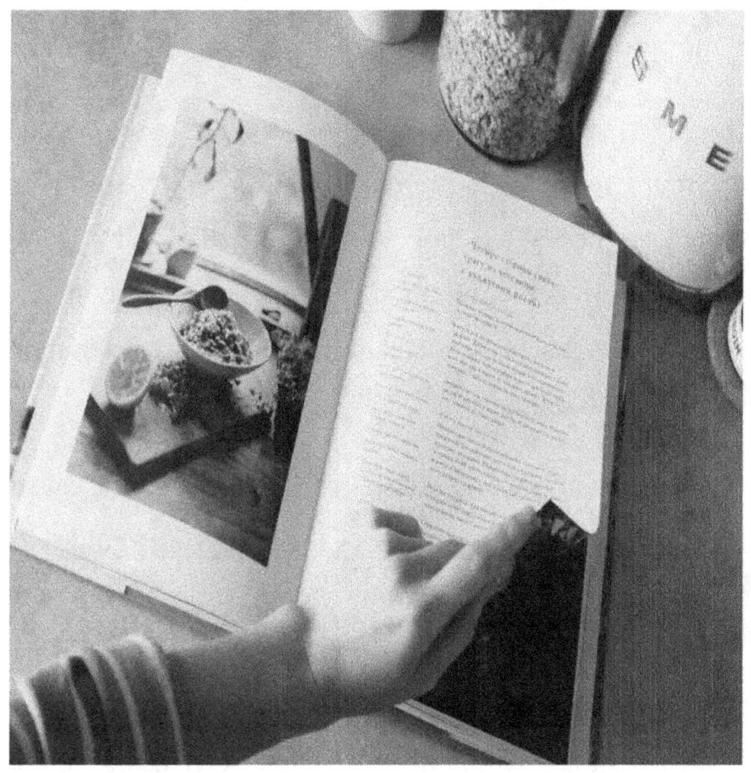

In the next chapter, we'll delve deeper into the prevalence of histamine intolerance, exploring its estimated numbers and the challenges in diagnosis. With this knowledge, we can better navigate the world of histamine and create a path towards a healthier, more enjoyable life.

The prevalence of histamine intolerance

Histamine - it's the term that appears like a naughty jester in the lives of many people dealing with a symphony of perplexing symptoms. Headaches that tap dance on your forehead, a gut that throws a tantrum after a seemingly harmless meal, and weariness that makes climbing Mount Everest look like a walk in the park are just a few notes in the discordant symphony of histamine intolerance. But here's the startling twist: unlike a traditional allergy, when a war cry is issued against a recognizable adversary (such as pollen or peanuts), histamine intolerance is a more subtle opponent.

So, how pervasive is this histamine craze? While determining exact statistics can be difficult, some estimates imply that histamine intolerance affects 1-3% of the general population. Consider this: there might be millions of individuals suffering from this mysterious ailment all across the world.

Diagnosis is an important aspect of the difficulty. Unlike a blood test, which may conclusively indicate an allergy, there is no single, definitive test for histamine intolerance. It's more like piecing together a detective tale by examining your symptoms, food triggers, and reaction to a histamine-free elimination diet. The good news is that, while diagnosing the ailment may need more investigation, there are effective management techniques available.

Now, you may be wondering why some of us are more sensitive to the histamine rush. Prepare to be enthralled by Chapter 2's exploration of genetics and enzymes. We'll look at how our genetics influence how our bodies manufacture and degrade histamine, as well as the importance of enzymes like diamine oxidase (DAO), the body's devoted "histamine disposal crew." Understanding these characteristics explains why some people have more intense symptoms than others.

But here's the most important takeaway

There is hope, regardless of the prevalence or cause of your sensitivity. This book is your guide to navigating the histamine world with confidence. We'll teach you how to recognize triggers, explore tasty low-histamine meals, and find strategies to improve your general health. So, let's change the page and rewrite the tale of histamine intolerance, from a tedious symphony to a victorious gastronomic journey!

THE ROLE OF GENETICS AND ENZYMES

How genetics influence histamine breakdown

Histamine intolerance might sometimes feel like a cosmic joke. You enjoy a meal, entirely innocent of any crime, and your body throws a fit. However, our inclination to respond to histamine may have deep genetic roots.

Think of your genes as the blueprints for your body. They influence everything from your eye color to your susceptibility to numerous diseases. When it comes to histamine, certain genes encode enzymes responsible for its breakdown. The enzyme diamine oxidase, or DAO for short, plays a very crucial role in this scenario. Consider DAO as your body's "histamine disposal crew." It degrades histamine in the intestines, keeping levels under control.

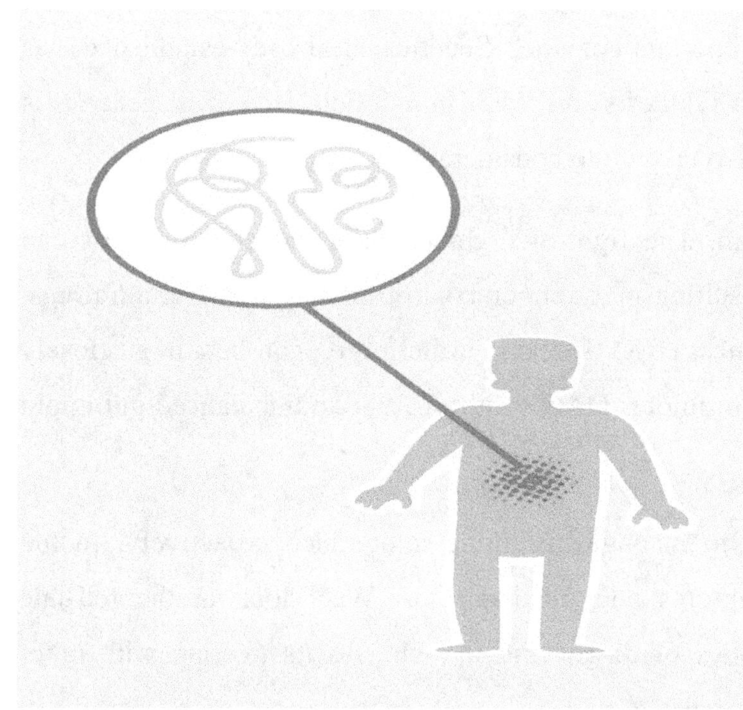

This is where the genetic story twist comes in. Some people inherit genetic variants that code for DAO. These changes can cause a reduction in DAO synthesis, making it more difficult for the body to break down histamine efficiently. This diminished activity produces a perfect storm for histamine intolerance, a condition in which even moderate doses of histamine cause symptoms.

However, genetics alone cannot provide the entire tale. Environmental conditions can also alter DAO activity. Stress, certain drugs, and even gut health may all make a difference.

In the following chapter, we'll go further into the interesting realm of diamine oxidase (DAO). We'll look at its critical role in histamine breakdown, how it may be impacted, and various strategies to help it work. Understanding DAO is critical for controlling histamine intolerance and creating a plan for a healthy you. So, keep reading to discover the mysteries of DAO and its influence on your well-being!

The importance of diamine oxidase (DAO)

Consider a little superhero patrolling your digestive tract, carrying the ability to neutralize a naughty foe: histamine. This enzyme, appropriately termed diamine oxidase (DAO), is essential for regulating histamine levels. Understanding its value is critical for navigating the world of histamine intolerance.

DAO is an enzyme that is largely generated in the gut, especially the small intestinal lining. It serves as the body's devoted "histamine disposal crew," meticulously breaking down histamine from meals and keeping it from wreaking havoc.

When DAO works adequately, it effectively neutralizes histamine, resulting in a smooth digestive symphony. When DAO function is impaired, even moderate quantities of histamine can overwhelm the system, resulting in the discordant notes of histamine intolerance - headaches, lethargy, digestive problems, and a slew of other undesirable symptoms.

So, what might interfere with the action of this important enzyme? Genetics, as already established, has a role. Variations in the genes involved for DAO synthesis can result in a deficit. However, genetics is not the only cause. Environmental elements are also taken into consideration.

Stress, for example, may become a DAO villain. The fight-or-flight reaction induced by stress can redirect resources away from DAO synthesis, resulting in a temporary drop in activity. Certain drugs, such as antidepressants, can potentially influence DAO levels. Furthermore, gut health is closely connected to DAO function. A healthy gut flora promotes DAO synthesis, but an unbalanced gut might lead to its reduction.

Understanding these characteristics allows you to manage histamine intolerance proactively. In the following chapter, we'll look at common symptoms and misdiagnoses. We'll look at the tell-tale indicators of histamine intolerance, the difficulties of diagnosing it owing to its overlap with other illnesses, and tactics for distinguishing it from allergies.

<u>But here's the most important takeaway:</u> DAO is your body's primary defense against histamine excess. You may improve your health and manage histamine intolerance by supporting its function and reducing things that interfere with it. Continue reading to learn how to confidently navigate the world of histamine!

COMMON SYMPTOMS AND MISDIAGNOSES

Identifying histamine-related symptoms

Histamine intolerance might feel like a disjointed symphony of symptoms, leaving you wondering what's going on inside your body. Headaches beat a persistent rhythm, your belly churns forth a chaotic solo, and exhaustion throws a heavy blanket over your entire body. Identifying histamine-related symptoms, however, is the first step in restoring balance in your health.

The most frequent symptom of histamine intolerance is stomach discomfort. Consider a churning, cramping sensation in your stomach following a seemingly benign meal. Bloating, gas, and even diarrhea are all symptoms of histamine causing havoc in your digestive tract.

Headaches, especially migraines, are another common cause. Histamine can cause vasodilation (widening of blood vessels) in the brain, resulting in throbbing discomfort and a pulsing feeling. Skin problems enter the list of symptoms. Itchy rashes, hives, and flushing (redness on the face or neck) are all symptoms of histamine intolerance.

But here's the catch: these symptoms frequently coincide with other illnesses, posing a diagnostic challenge. Fatigue, for example, can be a sign of a variety of conditions, including stress and anemia. Similarly, headaches can be caused by a number of circumstances. This is why the following chapter, Distinguishing Between Allergies and Intolerance, is essential.

We'll look at the fundamental differences between histamine allergy and intolerance, so you can appreciate the subtleties of their responses. We'll also talk about the difficulties of diagnosing and ways for getting a better understanding of what's causing your symptoms.

However, here's a useful beginning point: maintaining a food journal may be an investigator's best friend. By methodically recording what you consume and noting any following symptoms, you may discover possible triggers and begin developing a specific strategy for controlling histamine intolerance.

Don't be disheartened by the array of symptoms. Remember that recognizing histamine-related symptoms is the first step toward achieving harmony of well-being. With information as your weapon and tasty low-histamine recipes at your disposal, you can rewrite the symphony of your health and rediscover your love of food!

Differentiating between allergies and intolerance

Consider two wicked individuals producing comparable havoc in your body: allergies and histamine intolerance. Both can cause annoying symptoms such as headaches, exhaustion, and stomach problems, making it difficult to determine the exact reason. But don't worry; recognizing the essential distinctions between these two opponents will allow you to confidently traverse the world of histamine.

Allergies trigger a full-blown immune system reaction. When you encounter an allergen (such as pollen or peanuts), your immune system misidentifies it as a threat and initiates a counterattack. This causes the production of histamine and other inflammatory molecules, resulting in the characteristic allergy symptoms of runny nose, sneezing, and itchy eyes. The response is often quick and involves a specific allergy.

Histamine intolerance, on the other hand, does not trigger a full-fledged immunological response. It's more of a case of overwhelm. Your body may have trouble breaking down histamine owing to factors such as low DAO activity or intestinal abnormalities. This causes a buildup of histamine, which can produce symptoms similar to allergies but with several crucial differences.

The timing is one hint. Allergic responses are usually quick, happening within minutes of exposure to the allergen. Histamine intolerance symptoms, on the other hand, may take hours or even days to appear. The amount is also an important consideration. Allergies frequently exhibit a definite dose-response connection, with a higher quantity of the allergen causing a more severe reaction. However, histamine intolerance symptoms can be produced by relatively insignificant quantities of histamine, and the severity varies according to individual tolerance levels.

Diagnosis is another distinguishing feature. Allergy testing can identify the precise allergens causing your response. While there is no one reliable test for histamine intolerance, elimination diets and symptoms might give useful information.

Finding successful management solutions requires identifying the source of the problem, whether it be an allergy or intolerance. In the following chapter, we will look at the Gut Connection. We'll look at how your gut health affects histamine metabolism and explain how to create a gut environment that promotes healthy histamine breakdown. . So, keep reading to discover the secrets of regulating histamine for a life full of tasty food and healthy health!

THE GUT CONNECTION

Exploring the link between gut health and histamine intolerance

Imagine your gut as a busy metropolis filled with billions of microscopic people known as your gut microbiome. These tiny inhabitants play important roles in digestion, immunity, and even mood. However, their effect goes much farther, altering how your body manages histamine, the perplexing chemical at the core of intolerance. Understanding the gut connection is critical to managing your histamine journey.

A healthy gut microbiome supports friendly bacteria that aid in the breakdown of histamine from meals. These helpful microorganisms serve as your own "histamine disposal crew," guaranteeing proper digestion and keeping histamine levels under control. However, when the gut environment becomes unbalanced, with an invasion of "bad" bacteria, things might get worse.

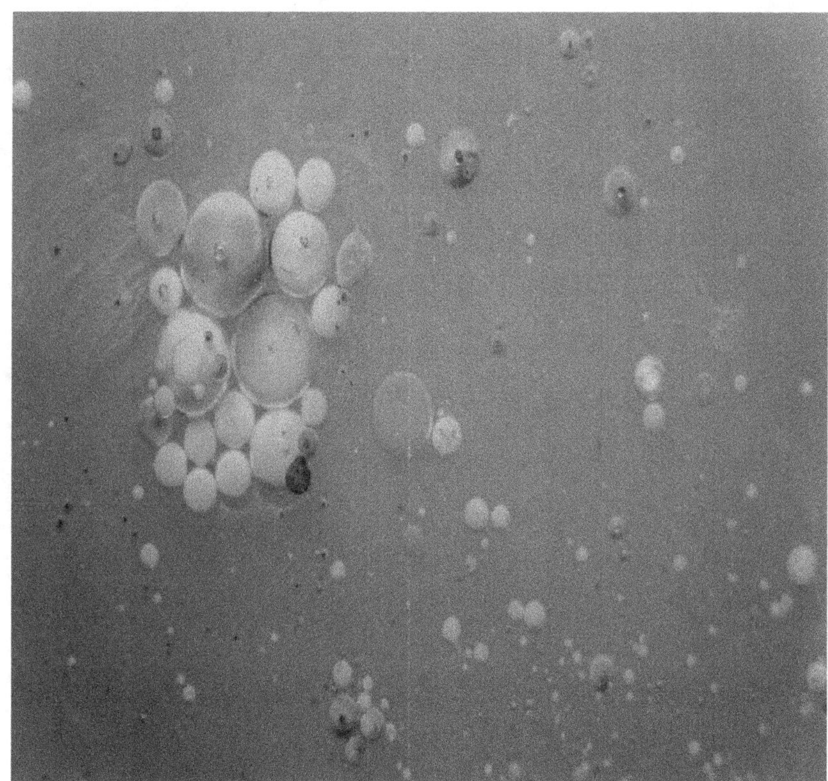

This imbalance, known as dysbiosis, can interfere with the gut's normal breakdown of histamines. Furthermore, inflammation in the gut lining, a typical side effect of dysbiosis, might decrease DAO synthesis, the enzyme responsible for further breaking down histamine. This perfect storm of decreased breakdown and higher histamine levels might produce the unpleasant symphony of symptoms associated with intolerance.

But here's the good news: the gut microbiota is extremely adaptive. You may cultivate a healthy gut environment by applying dietary and lifestyle recommendations that promote beneficial bacteria development and adequate histamine breakdown.

In the following chapter, we will look at how to implement dietary and lifestyle strategies to support gut health. We will look at particular dietary modifications, probiotics, and lifestyle behaviors that can help restore balance to your gut flora and provide the groundwork for improved histamine control.

Remember that a healthy gut is a happy gut, which implies a simpler road through histamine intolerance. Nurturing your gut environment allows your body to better tolerate histamine, paving the path for a more vigorous and pleasant existence. So, continue reading to discover the power of your stomach for a healthier you!

Implementing dietary and lifestyle strategies to support a healthy gut

When your gut flora is in good health, it might resemble a dynamic symphony performing in perfect harmony. But, like any symphony, a healthy stomach requires a good conductor, and you hold the baton! You may cultivate a healthy gut ecology by applying dietary and lifestyle recommendations, which promote optimum histamine breakdown and provide the framework for better histamine control.

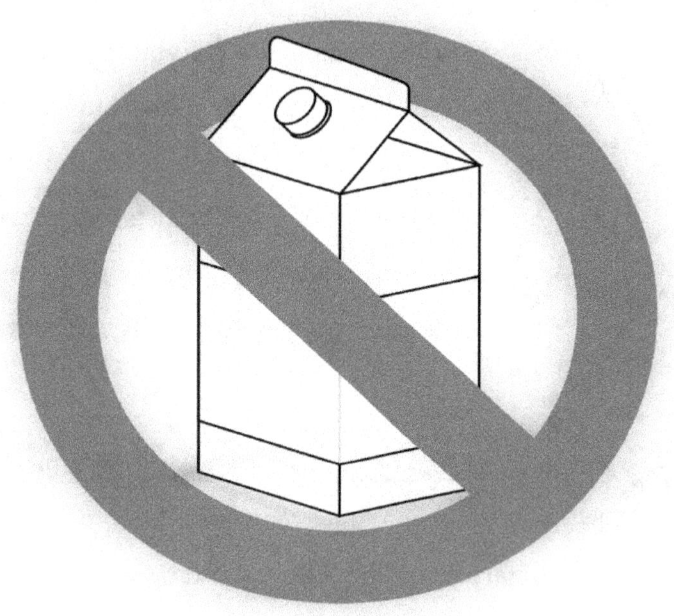

Dietary choices are the foundation of a gut-supportive strategy. Prioritize prebiotic-rich meals, which provide "fuel" for healthy bacteria in your gut. Think about colorful fruits and vegetables, lentils, and whole grains. Consider adding fermented foods such as yogurt, kimchi, and kefir, which are a natural source of probiotics, friendly bacteria that assist with digestion and histamine breakdown.

Fiber, your gut's "broom," also plays an important role. Adequate fiber consumption helps food pass more smoothly through your digestive tract, minimizing histamine buildup and its potential to cause problems. Choose whole grains, fruits with peel, and vegetables over processed carbs, which can lead to intestinal dysbiosis.

Hydration is a quiet maestro that keeps your gut symphony in tune. Water is necessary for proper digestion and maintains the integrity of your gut lining, limiting histamine leaks into the circulation. Aim for eight glasses of water each day, and adapt according to your activity level.

Lifestyle changes, in addition to diet, can have a significant impact on gut health. Stress upsets the delicate equilibrium in your stomach, therefore stress-reduction activities such as yoga or meditation may be quite useful. Sleep is another important factor; getting enough sleep helps your gut to relax and heal, which improves its function.

In the following chapter, "High-Histamine Culprits: Foods to Avoid," we'll look more closely at which foods contain high quantities of histamine or cause its production. We'll put together a complete list of items to avoid, allowing you to make informed dietary decisions and confidently manage your histamine journey.

A healthy stomach is the cornerstone for your overall health. By applying these tactics and making mindful dietary changes, you may create a healthy gut flora that effectively processes histamine, opening the door to a world of delicious food and robust well-being. So, continue reading to discover the power of your stomach for a healthier you!

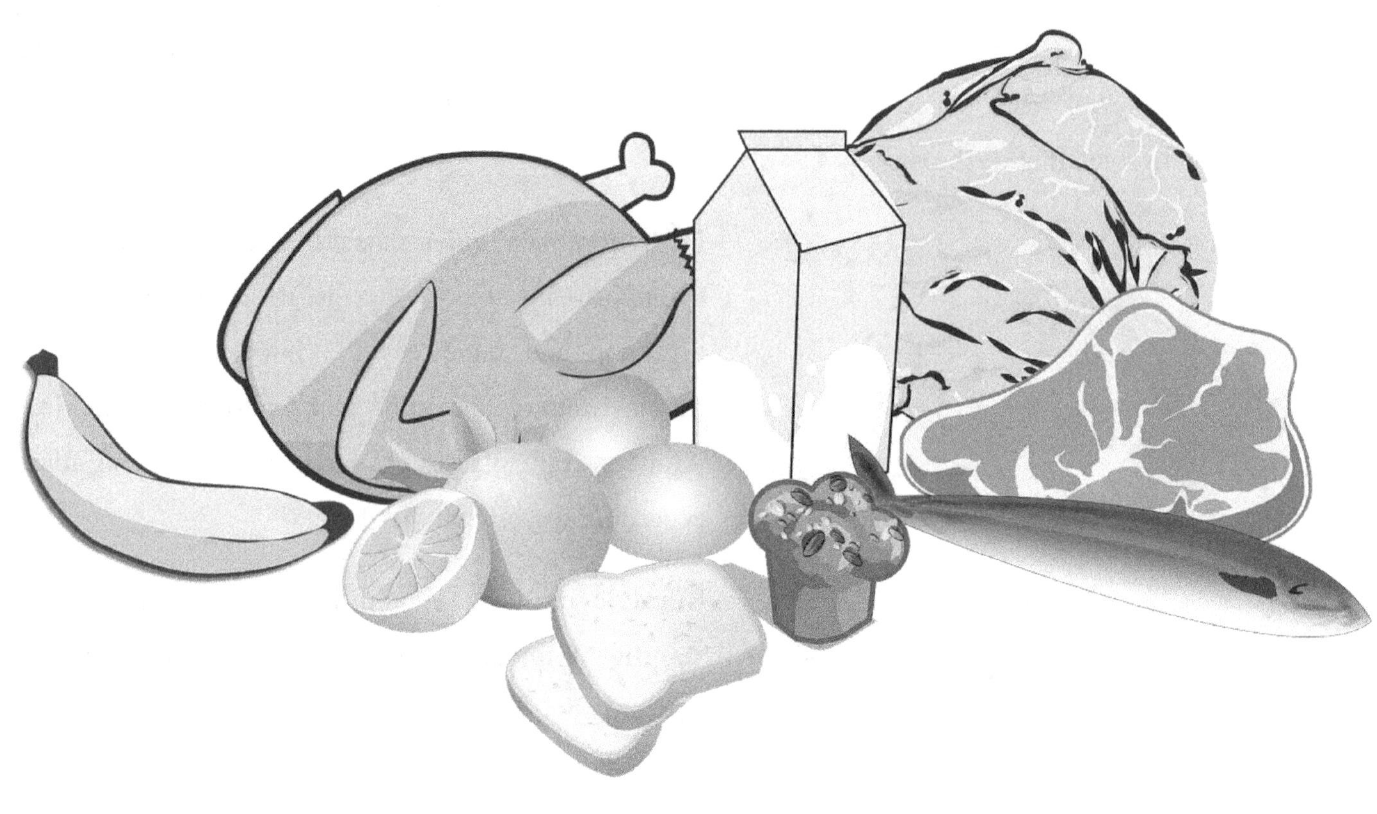

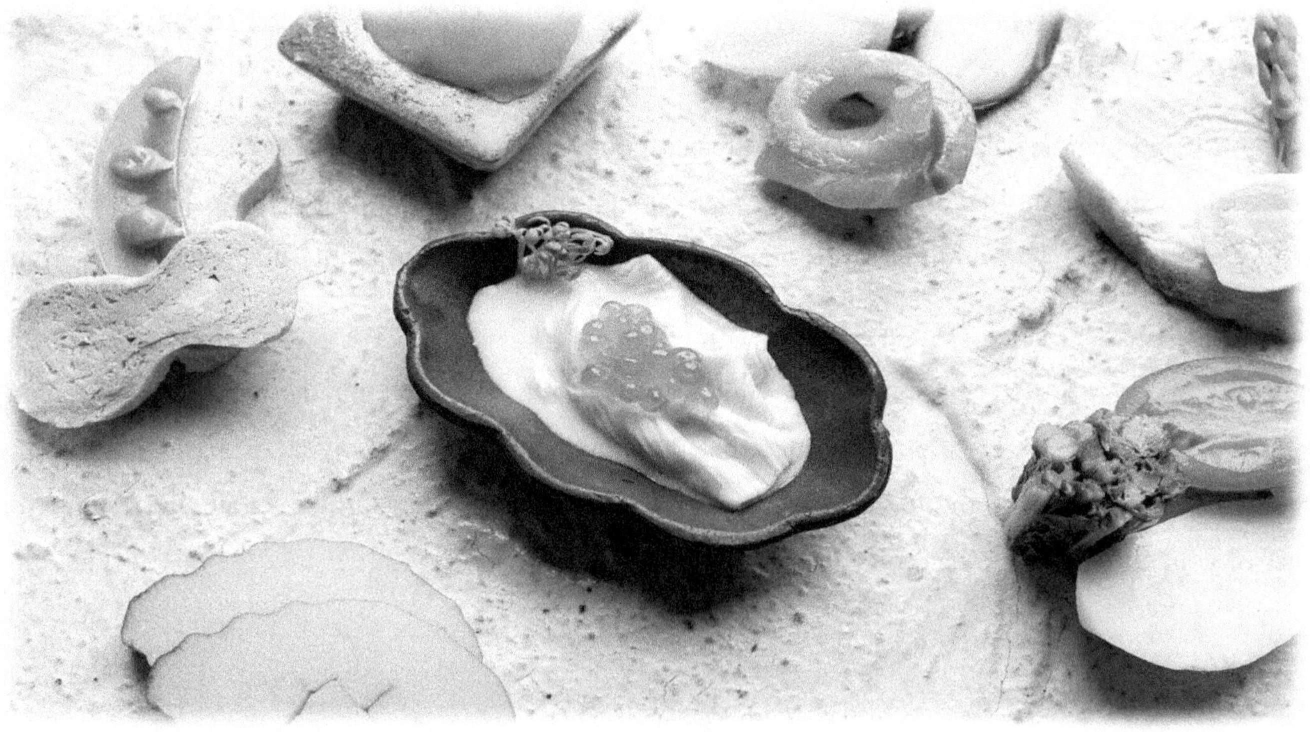

HIGH-HISTAMINE CULPRITS: FOODS TO AVOID

Fermented foods, aged cheeses, and alcohol

If you have histamine intolerance, it might be difficult to navigate the food world. Fermented foods, aged cheeses, and alcohol are three groups with very high histamine levels. Understanding these concepts and making educated decisions might help you manage your diet more effectively.

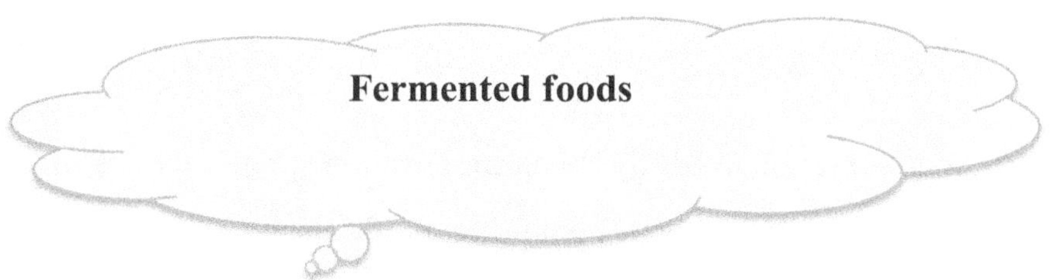

Fermentation, a process involving bacterial cultures, enhances the flavor and nutritional value of foods. However, it also produces histamines. While certain fermented foods, such as yogurt, may be tolerated in modest quantities, others provide a bigger issue. Here's what to look out for:

Sauerkraut and Kimchi: These famous fermented veggies are known for their high histamine content.

Kefir and Kombucha are popular fermented drinks that can cause histamine responses, particularly in unpasteurized variants. Choose low-histamine options, such as water kefir.

Sourdough Bread: While some studies indicate that sourdough may be better accepted than ordinary bread, proceed with caution and watch your body's reaction.

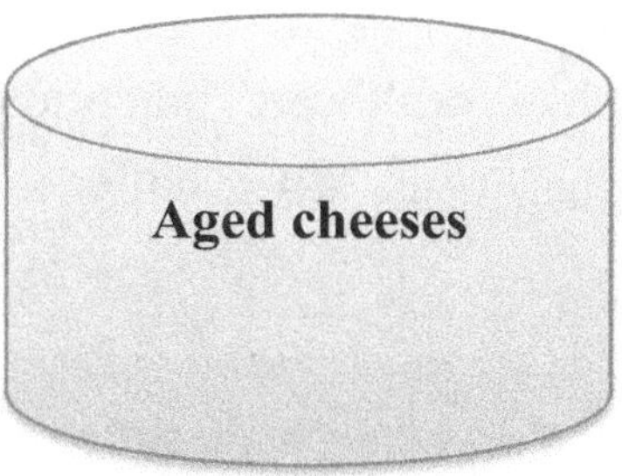

Cheese's aging process causes microorganisms to break down proteins, which increases histamine levels. In general, aged cheese has a greater histamine concentration. Some cheeses to avoid are:

Hard cheeses include Parmesan, Cheddar, Romano, and Blue. Cheeses: Gorgonzola and Roquefort

Soft-ripened cheeses: Brie and Camembert

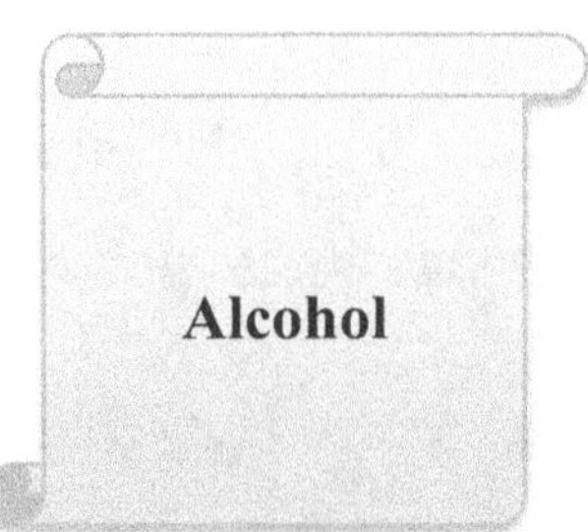

Some people's sensitivity to alcohol is caused by histamine rather than alcohol itself. Alcoholic beverages commonly contain significant quantities of histamine, particularly:

Wine: Red wine has more histamine than white.

Beer's histamine levels fluctuate based on the kind and brewing procedure.

Spirits: Although histamine levels are normally low, some persons respond.

Navigating these high-histamine foods

Begin with an Elimination Diet: Consult a healthcare practitioner to determine your individual triggers. This entails avoiding high-histamine meals for a while before gradually returning them to measure responses.

Fresh Is Best: Choose fresh, unprocessed meals whenever feasible.

Read labels carefully. Look for fermented foods in unexpected places, such as salad dressings and sauces.

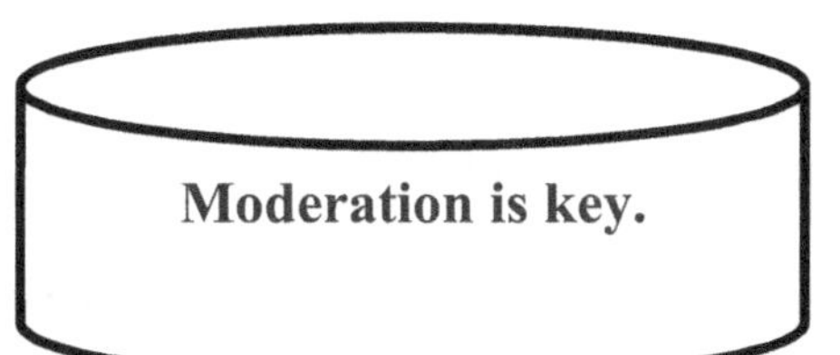

Even fermented foods with modest histamine levels might create issues if ingested in excess.

Beyond the obvious offenders, numerous seemingly innocent foods can contain hidden histamine. In the following chapter, we'll look deeper into these surprising sources, allowing you to make informed food choices while managing histamine sensitivity.

Reading food labels effectively

For people with histamine intolerance, browsing the grocery store might feel like decoding a hidden code. Food labels, while relatively simple, can include hidden sources of histamine. However, with a sharp eye and the correct understanding, you may convert them into strong instruments for optimal nutrition management.

Know Your Enemy: Histamine and Its Liberators

There are two primary offenders to look out for on food labels.

Histamine: This naturally occurring chemical found in some meals might directly cause intolerance symptoms.

Histamine Liberators: These are nutrients that cause your body to produce its own histamine, even if the food itself contains little.

Focus on the Ingredients List

The ingredient list on a food label serves as a route map. The ingredients are given in descending order of amount, with the most prominent component appearing first. Here's what you should look for:

High-Histamine Foods: Be mindful of histamine-rich foods, such as old cheeses (Parmesan, cheddar), fermented items (sauerkraut, kimchi), some fish (tuna, mackerel), and processed meats.

Histamine Liberators: Scan for chemicals that might cause your body to release histamines. Citrus fruits, tomatoes, spinach, avocado, nuts (cashews, peanuts), and food additives (MSG, nitrates, nitrites) are all common causes.

Beyond the Ingredient List

While the components list is important, other information on the label might be useful:

Freshness Indicators: Choose fresh, unprocessed meals wherever feasible. Look for "sell by" or "use by" dates to get the freshest selections.

Processing methods: Be aware of how food is prepared. Fermentation, drying, and aging all raise histamine levels. Look for minimally processed alternatives.

Hidden histamine in unexpected places: Histamine can appear in unexpected areas. Check the ingredients in condiments, dressings, sauces, and even prepared meals. Avoid broad phrases like "spices" or "natural flavors" since they may contain histamine liberators.

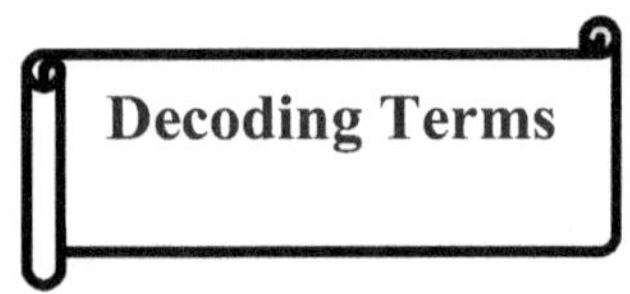

The phrases "naturally occurring" or "bio-identical" do not ensure that a meal is low in histamine. Histamine is found naturally in many foods.

"Low-Sodium" or "Reduced Sodium" labels may appear healthful, but some manufacturers replace salt with nitrates or nitrites, which can be histamine liberators.

Overnight Oats

Ingredients

1/2 cup rolled oats (old-fashioned oats are ideal)

3/4 cup nondairy milk (such as almond, coconut, or hemp milk).

1 tablespoon of chia seeds (optional for extra texture and nutrients).

1 tablespoon maple syrup (for sweetness).

1/4 teaspoon of vanilla extract (optional for taste).

Fresh fruits, such as blueberries, apples, or mangoes.

Nuts and seeds (almonds or flaxseeds, if permitted)

Preparation

Combine rolled oats, non-dairy milk, chia seeds, maple syrup, and vanilla essence in a mason jar or dish.

Stir Well: Make sure all of the ingredients are thoroughly incorporated.

Refrigerate the jar or bowl overnight (at least 6-8 hours).

Toppings: In the morning, mix the oats well. Top with your favorite fresh fruits and nuts/seeds.

Serve your overnight oats directly from the container or transfer to a bowl.

Prep Time

Preparation takes 5 minutes.

Refrigeration: 6 to 8 hours (overnight)

Quinoa Porridge

Ingredients

4 tablespoons quinoa.

To make the recipe, combine 1/3 cup water and 1/4 cup coconut milk (free of gums and thickeners).

1 teaspoon honey, if acceptable.

1/2 cup of fresh blueberries.

Preparation

Rinse Quinoa well with cool water to eliminate any bitterness.

Cook Quinoa: In a small saucepan, mix the quinoa with the water. Bring to a boil, then lower to a simmer for 10-15 minutes, or until the water has virtually evaporated.

Stir in the coconut milk and continue cooking until the quinoa is mushy and has absorbed the majority of the liquid.

Sweetening: Remove from heat and mix in honey (if using).

Serve: Top with fresh blueberries and serve immediately.

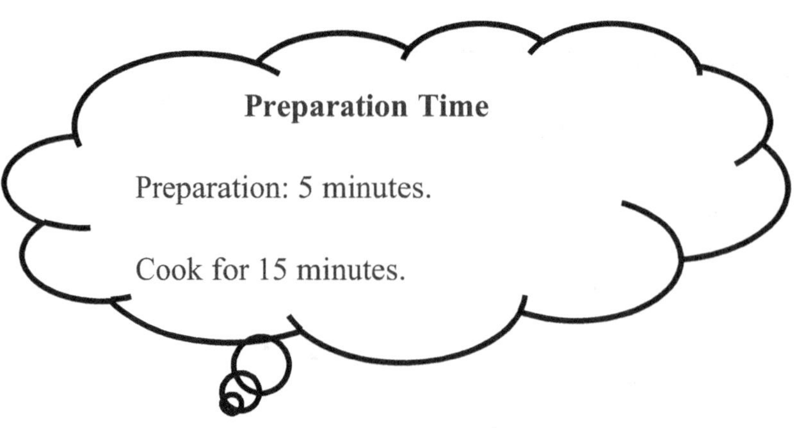

Buckwheat Pancakes

Ingredients

1 cup buckwheat flour.

1 tablespoon of baking powder.

Ingredients: 1/4 teaspoon salt, 1 cup water (or non-dairy milk, such as coconut or almond milk).

1 tablespoon of maple syrup (for sweetness)

1 teaspoon of vanilla extract (optional).

Coconut oil (for cooking).

Preparation

Dry Ingredients: In a large basin, combine the buckwheat flour, baking powder, and salt.

Wet ingredients: Combine the water (or non-dairy milk), maple syrup, and vanilla extract with the dry ingredients. Mix until barely mixed; the batter should be somewhat lumpy.

Heat Pan: Place a nonstick pan or griddle over medium heat and gently coat with coconut oil.

Cook Pancakes: Pour 1/4 cup batter into the skillet for each pancake. Cook for approximately 2-3 minutes, or until bubbles form on the surface and the edges seem firm. Flip and heat for a further 1-2 minutes, or until golden brown.

Serve warm with fresh fruit, such as blueberries or apples, and a sprinkle of maple syrup, if preferred.

Preparation Time

Preparation: 5 minutes.

Cook for 10 minutes.

Ingredients

Two big sweet potatoes, peeled and chopped

Dice 1 red bell pepper

1 yellow bell pepper

1 tiny white onion, and

2 tablespoons olive oil (low histamine content).

1/2 teaspoon of sea salt.

1/4 teaspoon black pepper (optional and if acceptable)

For garnish, use fresh herbs such as parsley or cilantro.

Preparation

Preheat oven to 400 degrees Fahrenheit (200 degrees Celsius).

Prepare vegetables: In a large mixing dish, add the diced sweet potatoes, bell peppers, and onion.

Season and toss: Drizzle with olive oil and season with sea salt and black pepper (if desired). Toss to coat evenly.

Roast Vegetables: Place the mixture in a single layer on a baking sheet. Roast the sweet potatoes in a preheated oven for 25-30 minutes, tossing halfway through, until soft and slightly crispy.

Serve: Remove from the oven and top with fresh herbs. Serve warm.

Preparation Time

Preparation: 10 minutes.

Cook for 25-30 minutes.

Chia Seed Pudding

Ingredients

1 cup nondairy milk (such as coconut or macadamia milk)

3 tablespoons chia seeds.

1 tablespoon flaxseed meal (optional for extra fiber)

1 teaspoon of vanilla powder or essence.

1-2 tablespoons maple syrup or honey (to taste)

Fresh fruit (e.g., blueberries, pears) for topping.

Preparation

Mix Ingredients: In a mixing dish or jar, combine the non-dairy milk, chia seeds, flaxseed meal (if using), vanilla, and sugar. Stir thoroughly to ensure that the chia seeds are uniformly dispersed.

Refrigerate: Cover the bowl or container and chill for at least 4 hours, or overnight. This causes the chia seeds to absorb the liquid and create a pudding-like texture.

Stir again. After the initial refrigeration, whisk the liquid thoroughly to break up any clumps.

Serve: Once the pudding has set, top with your favorite fresh fruit. Enjoy!

Preparation time

Activity time: 5 minutes

Chill time: four hours (or overnight).

Rice Cakes with Avocado

Ingredients

2 rice cakes (ideally prepared with brown rice)

1 ripe avocado.

1 teaspoon of lemon juice (optional, if tolerated).

Salt to taste.

Garnish with fresh herbs, such as parsley or cilantro.

Preparation

Prepare the Avocado: Cut the avocado in half, remove the pit, and scoop the flesh into a dish. Mash with a fork until smooth. If you tolerate lemon juice, mix some into the mashed avocado to avoid browning and provide some flavor.

Season the mashed avocado with a touch of salt and combine thoroughly.

Assemble by spreading the mashed avocado evenly over the rice cakes.

Garnish with fresh herbs to enhance taste and color.

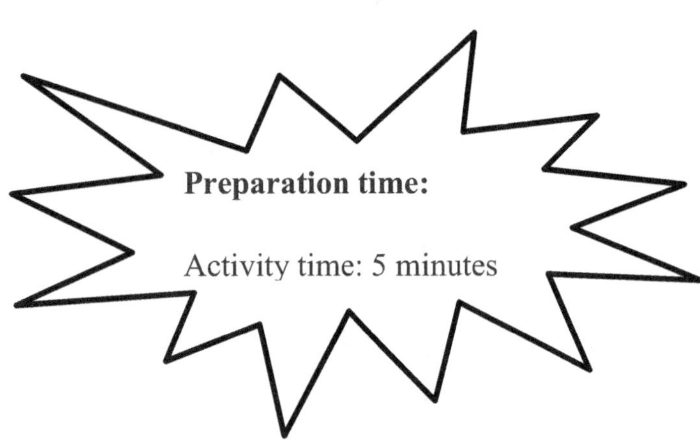

Millet Porridge

Ingredients

1 cup millet.

2 glasses of water.

1 cup nondairy milk (such as coconut or almond milk)

1 teaspoon of vanilla extract (optional).

1 tablespoon maple syrup or honey (to taste)

Fresh fruit (e.g., blueberries, pears) for topping.

Pinch of salt.

Preparation

Rinse Millet well with cold water to eliminate any contaminants.

Cook millet: In a medium saucepan, mix the washed millet with water and a pinch of salt. Bring to a boil over medium high heat.

Simmer: Once boiling, decrease the heat to low, cover, and allow it cook for approximately 20 minutes, or until the millet is soft and the water has been absorbed.

Add milk and sweetener. Combine the nondairy milk, vanilla extract (if using), and maple syrup or honey. Cook for another 5-10 minutes, stirring regularly, until the porridge is the appropriate consistency.

Serve by spooning the porridge into bowls and topping with fresh fruit of your choice.

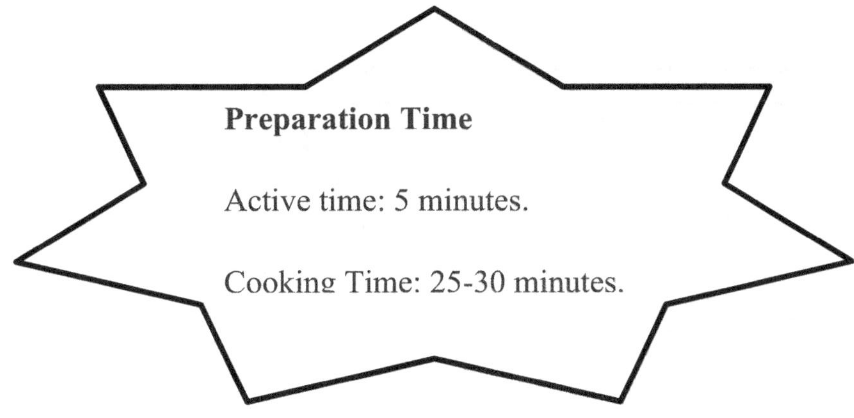

Coconut Yogurt Parfait

Ingredients

1 cup coconut yogurt (check it has histamine-friendly probiotics).

1/2 cup fresh berries (such as blueberries and raspberries)

1 tablespoon of chia seeds.

1 tablespoon flaxseed meal (optional for extra fiber)

1 tablespoon maple syrup or honey (to taste)

1/4 cup granola (make sure it's low in histamine and devoid of nuts and dried fruits).

Fresh mint leaves for garnish (optional).

Preparation

Layer the ingredients in a glass or dish, beginning with a layer of coconut yogurt.

Add toppings: Sprinkle fresh berries, chia seeds, and flaxseed meal (if using) on top of the yogurt.

To sweeten, drizzle with maple syrup or honey.

Repeat Layers: Add another layer of coconut yogurt, then additional berries, chia seeds, and flaxseed meal.

Top with granola. Finish with a layer of granola and some fresh mint leaves for garnish.

Preparation time

Active time: 10 minutes.

Apple Cinnamon Muffins

Ingredients

1 1/2 cups buckwheat flour.

1/2 cup rice or oat milk.

One tablespoon of lemon juice or apple cider vinegar

One medium apple, peeled and diced

1/4 cup maple syrup.

1/4 cup olive or coconut oil.

2 eggs

1 tablespoon ground flaxseed.

1 teaspoon baking powder (gluten-free).

1/2 teaspoon baking soda.

1/4 tsp salt, 1 tsp ground ginger (optional as a replacement for cinnamon).

Preparation Time
Preparation: 15 minutes.
Bake for 25-30 minutes.

Preparation

Preheat the oven to 180°C (350°F) and prepare a 12-hole muffin tray with paper liners.

Prepare the buttermilk: Combine the rice milk and lemon juice (or apple cider vinegar) to make a buttermilk alternative. Set aside.

Dry ingredients: In a large mixing bowl, add buckwheat flour, powdered flaxseed, baking powder, baking soda, and salt.

In another dish, combine the eggs, maple syrup, olive oil, and buttermilk mixture.

Combine Ingredients: Make a well in the center of the dry ingredients and pour in the wet mixture. Stir just until mixed.

Add apples: Fold in the diced apples lightly.

Fill the Muffin Tray: Distribute the batter evenly among the muffin cases.

Bake for 25-30 minutes, or until a toothpick inserted into the middle of each muffin comes out clean.

Cool: Let the muffins cool on the tray for 5 minutes before transferring to a wire rack to finish cooling.

Egg-Free Scramble

Ingredients

1 block firm tofu (fresh, not fermented)

1/2 cup chopped bell peppers, red or yellow.

1/2 cup chopped zucchini.

1/4 cup chopped green onions.

1 tablespoon olive oil.

1/2 teaspoon turmeric powder (for coloring)

1/2 teaspoon ground ginger (optional for flavoring)

Add salt and pepper to taste.

Fresh cilantro or parsley for garnish.

Preparation Time:

Preparation: 10 minutes.

Cooking time: 10-12 minutes.

Total: around 20-22 minutes.

Preparation

Prepare the tofu: Drain the tofu and dry it with a paper towel. Crumble it into little bits that resemble scrambled eggs.

Cook the vegetables: Heat the olive oil in a nonstick skillet over medium heat. Combine the chopped bell peppers, zucchini, and green onions. Sauté the veggies for about 5 minutes, until they are soft.

Add tofu and spices. Add the crushed tofu to the skillet. Season with turmeric powder, powdered ginger (if using), salt, and pepper. Stir well to mix.

Cook the scramble. Cook for a further 5-7 minutes, stirring periodically, until the tofu is cooked through and slightly brown.

Remove from the heat and sprinkle with fresh parsley or cilantro. Serve warm.

Oat Milk Pancakes

Ingredients

1 1/2 cups oat flour (this may be made by mixing oats).

1 cup oat milk.

1 tablespoon of ground flaxseed (for flax egg)

2 1/2 tbsp water and

1 tbsp maple syrup.

1 tablespoon of olive or coconut oil.

1 teaspoon baking powder (gluten-free).

1/2 teaspoon baking soda.

1/4 tsp salt

1/2 tsp ground ginger (optional for taste).

Preparation Time

Preparation: 10 minutes.

Cook for 15 minutes.

Total: around 25 minutes.

Preparation

Prepare the Flax Egg: In a small dish, combine the ground flaxseed and water. Allow it to settle for about 5 minutes, until it has a gel-like consistency.

Dry ingredients: In a large mixing bowl, combine oat flour, baking powder, baking soda, salt, and powdered ginger (if using).

In a separate dish, mix together the oat milk, flax egg, maple syrup, and olive oil.

Combine the ingredients by pouring the wet mixture into the dry and stirring until just incorporated. Allow the batter to sit for five minutes.

Cook the pancakes: Preheat a nonstick skillet over medium heat. Lightly grease with oil. Pour 1/4 cup batter each pancake onto the skillet. Cook until bubbles appear on the top, then turn and cook until golden brown on the opposite side.

Serve warm, with your favorite low histamine toppings, like as fresh fruit or maple syrup.

Blueberry Muffins

Ingredients

1 1/2 cups gluten-free flour blend.

1/2 cup coconut sugar or other low-histamine sweetener.

1/2 teaspoon salt

2 teaspoons baking powder (gluten-free).

2 teaspoons xanthan gum.

1/3 cup mild olive oil.

1 flax egg (1 tbsp of flaxseed + 2 1/2 tbsp of water)

1/3 cup water.

1 1/2 teaspoons vanilla extract (optional).

1 cup blueberries, fresh or frozen.

Preparation Time

Preparation: 10 minutes.

Bake for 12-15 minutes.

Total: around 25 minutes.

Preparation

Preheat the oven to 200°C (400°F) and coat a muffin tin with olive oil or line with paper cups.

Prepare the flax egg: In a small dish, combine the ground flaxseed and water. Allow it to settle for about 5 minutes, until it has a gel-like consistency.

Dry Ingredients: In a large mixing bowl, combine gluten-free flour blend, coconut sugar, salt, baking powder, and xanthan gum.

Mix Wet Ingredients: In a liquid measuring cup, add olive oil, flax egg, and water. If using, add the vanilla essence and whisk until thoroughly blended.

Combine the ingredients by pouring the wet mixture into the dry and stirring until just incorporated. The batter will be thick, so avoid overmixing.

Add Blueberries: Fold the blueberries into the muffin batter.

Fill Muffin Tray: Fill each muffin cup half to two-thirds full with batter.

Bake for 12-15 minutes for standard-sized muffins, or until a toothpick inserted into the center comes out clean.

Grilled Chicken Salad

Ingredients

Protein:

2 boneless, skinless chicken breasts (grilled or pan-seared).

Vegetables (all low histamine):

1 cup of diced cucumber.

1/2 cup of halved cherry tomatoes.

1/2 cup of diced red bell pepper.

1/4 cup crumbled feta cheese (optional; eliminate for a completely vegan version).

1/4 cup freshly chopped dill.

2 tablespoons of chopped fresh chives.

Low-Histamine Dressing:

3 tablespoons olive oil.

2 teaspoons of lemon juice.

1 tablespoon honey (or maple syrup as a vegan alternative)

1/2 teaspoon dried thyme.

1/4 teaspoon of garlic powder.

Add salt and freshly ground black pepper to taste.

Salad greens (choose low-histamine options):

A bed of arugula, baby spinach, or romaine lettuce

Preparation

(5 Minutes) Cook the chicken breasts on a hot grill or in a skillet with a little olive oil until well done. Let the chicken cool slightly before chopping or shredding it into bite-sized pieces.

(5 Minutes) While the chicken is cooking, prepare the veggies. Wash and cut the cucumber, cherry tomatoes, and red bell pepper. Finely cut the fresh dill and chives.

(5 Minutes) In a small jar or dish, combine the olive oil, lemon juice, honey, thyme, garlic powder, salt, and pepper to prepare the dressing.

(Assemble - 5 min) In a large mixing bowl, add the diced chicken, cucumber, cherry tomatoes, red bell pepper, feta cheese (if using), dill, and chives.

Pour the dressing over the salad and toss to coat evenly.

Serve the salad on a bed of low-histamine greens (romaine lettuce, baby spinach, or arugula are good options).

Quinoa and Vegetable Stir-Fry

Ingredients	**Preparation**

Ingredients

1 cup uncooked quinoa.

add 2 cups of water or low-sodium vegetable broth and

1 tablespoon of toasted or plain sesame oil.

1 tiny, chopped onion

Mince two cloves of garlic and one knob of fresh ginger.

2 cups broccoli florets.

1 small sliced bell pepper

2-3 julienned or sliced carrots,

4 oz. snow peas.

1 tablespoon of low-sodium soy sauce (or coconut aminos for a histamine-friendly option).

Optional: A sprinkle of red pepper flakes for spice (omit if sensitive).

To garnish, add white sesame seeds (optional).

Preparation

To cook the quinoa, first rinse it in cold water. In a saucepan, mix the quinoa and water (or broth). Bring to a boil, then decrease heat to low, cover, and cook for approximately 15 minutes, or until the quinoa is fluffy and the liquid has been absorbed.

To prepare the stir-fry, heat sesame oil in a large pan or wok over medium heat.

Combine the chopped onion, minced garlic, and ginger. Sauté for about 5 minutes, until the onion is transparent.

Place the broccoli, bell pepper, carrots, and snow peas in the pan. Cook for 5–7 minutes, stirring regularly, until the veggies are cooked but still crisp. If they begin to stick, use a spray of water.

Cook the veggies first, then add cooked quinoa to the pan. Stir well to mix.

Drizzle with low-sodium soy sauce (or coconut aminos) and mix well.

To serve, divide the stir-fry into dishes and top with sesame seeds as desired.

Turkey Lettuce Wraps

Ingredients

Turkey Breast Fillets: 2

Olive Oil: 1-2 teaspoons.

Chop 1 white onion and mince 2-3 garlic cloves.

Chop one bell pepper and one zucchini.

Fresh Ginger: 1 teaspoon grated.

Turmeric: One teaspoon

Apple juice: two teaspoons.

Lettuce Leaves: Large leaves (such as butter lettuce).

Tahini: two tablespoons.

Honey: one teaspoon.

Sesame seeds: 1 tablespoon for garnish.

Parsley: fresh, chopped, for garnish.

Prep time: 15 minutes.

Cook time: 15 minutes.

Total time: 30 minutes.

Instructions

Prepare the turkey: In a medium-size pan, heat the olive oil. Sauté the chopped onion and minced garlic until aromatic.

Cook the turkey: Place the turkey breast fillets in the skillet and cook until no longer pink. Shred the turkey with two forks.

Add Vegetables: Place the diced bell pepper and zucchini in the pan. Cook the veggies until they're soft.

Seasoning: Add the grated ginger and turmeric. To keep the mixture wet, add a dash of apple juice.

Prepare the lettuce wraps. Wash and dry the lettuce leaves. Arrange them on a serving plate.

Make the dressing: In a small bowl, combine the tahini, honey, and a pinch of fresh ginger. Drizzle it over the turkey mixture.

Assemble: Place the turkey and vegetable combination in the lettuce leaves. Garnish with sesame seeds and chopped parsley.

Serve: Enjoy your low histamine turkey lettuce wraps!

Sweet Potato and Kale Bowl

Ingredients

2 medium sweet potatoes, peeled and diced

1 tablespoon of olive oil.

1/2 teaspoon ground cumin

1/4 teaspoon smoked paprika.

Add sea salt and black pepper to taste.

4 cups chopped kale with stems removed.

1 cup cooked quinoa.

1/2 cup canned chickpeas, washed, drained

1/4 cup chopped green onions.

2 tablespoons of toasted pumpkin seeds.

1 tablespoon of lemon juice.

1 tablespoon of low-sodium soy sauce or coconut aminos.

Preparation

Preheat the oven to 400° F (200° C).

In a large mixing basin, combine the diced sweet potatoes, olive oil, cumin, paprika, salt, and pepper. Spread onto a baking sheet lined with parchment paper.

Roast sweet potatoes for 20-25 minutes, tossing halfway through, until soft and lightly browned. Set aside to cool somewhat.

Massage the chopped kale in a large mixing basin with lemon juice and soy sauce (or coconut aminos) until tender.

Combine the roasted sweet potatoes, cooked quinoa, chickpeas, green onions, and pumpkin seeds with the greens. Toss gently until combined.

Serve the sweet potato and kale dish warm or room temperature.

Preparation Time

Total preparation time: around 35 minutes.

Sweet potato roasting time is 20-25 minutes.

Kale Massage and Assembly: 10 minutes.

Chicken and Avocado Salad

Ingredients

Chicken breast: 2 fillets, cooked and shredded

Avocado: one big, diced

Cucumber: 1 diced

Red onion: 1/4 cup coarsely chopped.

Fresh cilantro: 2 teaspoons, chopped.

Olive oil: 2 teaspoons.

Lemon juice: one tablespoon.

Sea salt: to taste.

Black pepper to taste (optional).

Instructions

Cook the Chicken: If the chicken is not already cooked, season the fillets with a sprinkle of sea salt and black pepper. Cook the chicken in a pan over medium heat with a little olive oil until well done. Allow to cool and then shred.

Prepare the vegetables. While the chicken cooks, dice the avocado and cucumber, and finely cut the red onion and cilantro.

Mix the salad: In a large mixing bowl, add the shredded chicken, diced avocado, cucumber, red onion, and cilantro.

Make the dressing: In a small bowl, combine the olive oil and lemon juice. Pour it over the salad and gently toss to incorporate.

Season with sea salt and black pepper to taste.

Serve: Enjoy your fresh and nutritious low-histamine chicken and avocado salad!

Prep time: 15 minutes.

Cook for 10 minutes (if the chicken is not pre-cooked).

Total time: 25 minutes.

Butternut Squash Soup

Ingredient	**Preparation**

Ingredient

1 small butternut squash (about 2 pounds), peeled and diced

Halve 2-3 cloves of garlic (or ½ small onion if desired).

2 cups tolerated coconut milk or veggie broth.

½ teaspoon sea salt (modify depending on the saltiness of the broth).

1 tablespoon olive oil (or another suitable oil)

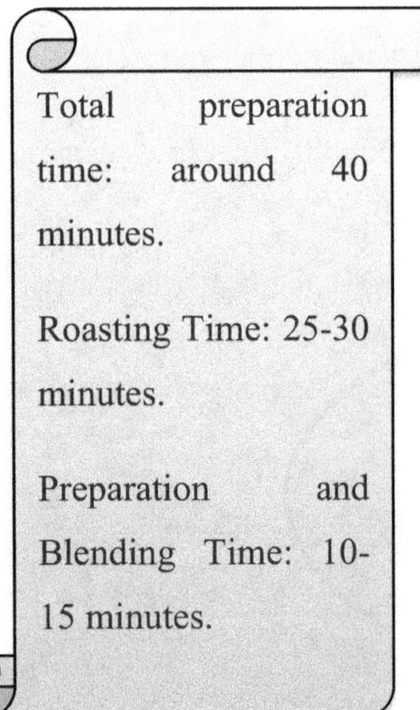

Preparation

Preheat the oven to 400°F (205°C).

Prepare the squash and garlic.

Peel and cube the butternut squash. Cut the garlic in half.

To prepare for roasting, combine cubed squash and garlic with olive oil and sea salt in a large bowl. Place them in a single layer on a baking sheet coated with parchment paper.

Roast the squash in a warm oven for 25-30 minutes, or until soft and beginning to color.

Blend the soup.

Let the roasted squash and garlic cool for a few minutes. Transfer to a big pot. Add the vegetable stock or coconut milk.

Using an immersion blender, puree the ingredients until smooth. Alternatively, you may mix in batches in a powerful blender.

If the soup is too thick, add more broth or coconut milk to achieve the required consistency.

To serve, ladle soup into bowls and enjoy warm. Optional garnishes include sesame seeds and a dollop of coconut cream.

Millet and Roasted Veggie Bowl

Ingredients

1 cup millet.

2 cups low-sodium vegetable broth.

One small butternut squash, peeled and cubed

Cut one red bell pepper

one zucchini

one small onion into slices.

2 tablespoons olive oil.

1 teaspoon ground cumin.

1/2 teaspoon of smoked paprika.

1/4 teaspoon of cayenne pepper (optional; omit if sensitive).

Add sea salt and black pepper to taste.

1-cup cooked chickpeas (optional)

2 tablespoons of toasted pumpkin seeds.

Lemon wedges for serving.

Preparation

To cook millet, combine it with vegetable broth and bring to a boil. Reduce the heat, cover, and cook for 20-25 minutes until done. Fluff with a fork, then set aside.

Roast the vegetables.

Preheat the oven to 400° F (200° C).

In a large mixing bowl, combine the cubed butternut squash, bell pepper, zucchini, and onion with olive oil, cumin, paprika, cayenne (if using), salt, and pepper.

Place the veggies on a baking sheet lined with parchment paper. Roast for 20-25 minutes, stirring halfway through, until soft and gently browned.

Assemble the bowls

Divide the cooked millet into serving cups.

Finish with roasted veggies, chickpeas (if using), and toasted pumpkin seeds.

Serve warm, with lemon wedges on the side to squeeze over top.

Total preparation time: around 50 minutes.

Millet Cook time: 20-25 minutes.

Vegetable roasting time: 20-25 minutes

Assembly time: five minutes.

Egg-Free Frittata

Ingredients	**Preparation**

Ingredients

3/4 cup split mung beans (moong dal washed)

1 ¼ teaspoon black salt (or sea salt).

1/2 teaspoon onion powder.

3/4 teaspoon ground turmeric.

1 ⅓ cups canned light coconut milk

2 tablespoons olive or avocado oil (plus more for cooking)

1/4 cup chickpea flour (white rice flour)

1 ¼ teaspoon baking powder

1 cup veggies (such as finely sliced red onion or slow-roasted tomatoes)

1/4 cup macadamia nut cheese (or any other soft vegan cheese).

Fresh herbs (dill, basil, or parsley; optional)

Vegan Parmesan Cheese (optional)

Preparation

Soak the Mung Beans: Rinse the split mung beans and transfer them to a large mixing dish. Cover with lukewarm water and soak for at least 6 hours, preferably overnight.

After soaking, rinse the mung beans and place them in a blender. Combine the black salt, onion powder, turmeric, coconut milk, olive oil, chickpea flour, and baking powder. Blend until smooth and creamy.

Prepare the pan: Preheat the oven to 375°F (190° C). Heat a little amount of olive oil in an oven-safe skillet (ideally cast iron) over medium heat.

Cook the Frittata: Transfer the mixed mixture to a heated skillet. Top with your preferred veggies and macadamia nut cheese. Optional toppings include fresh herbs and vegan Parmesan cheese.

Bake: Place the pan in the preheated oven for 25-30 minutes, or until the frittata is set and somewhat puffy.

Serve: Allow to cool somewhat before slicing. Serve warm or room temperature.

Cauliflower Rice Stir-Fry

Ingredients

1 head of cauliflower, {grated or shredded into "rice"}

1 tablespoon coconut oil (or water if you don't want to use oil).

1 ½ cups green beans, (trimmed and halved)

1 medium bell pepper, finely sliced (red, orange, or yellow)

1 cup sliced green onions (set aside some green tops for serving)

1 cup thinly sliced cabbage, either red or green.

1/4 cup roasted cashews, (or slivered toasted almonds)

2 tablespoons coconut aminos (to season)

1 tablespoon maple syrup (or coconut sugar, if you want)

1 tablespoon of minced fresh ginger (or 1/2 teaspoon powdered ginger).

2 tablespoons of lime juice.

Preparation

Prepare the Cauliflower Rice: Remove the cauliflower's green stalks and shred it using a box grater or food processor until it resembles rice. Set aside.

Heat the Oil: Place a large pan over medium heat and add the coconut oil (or water). Once hot, add the green beans and cook for about 4 minutes, stirring periodically.

Vegetables: Place the sliced bell pepper, green onions, and cabbage in the pan. Stir in the veggies and simmer for a further 3-4 minutes, or until just soft.

Incorporate Cauliflower Rice: Place the grated cauliflower rice in the pan with the roasted cashews. Stir well to combine all of the ingredients.

Make the Sauce: In a small dish, combine the coconut aminos, maple syrup, chopped ginger, and lime juice. Pour the sauce over the stir-fry ingredients in the skillet.

Increase the heat to medium-high and cook for another 3-5 minutes, stirring often, until everything is well cooked and well mixed.

Remove from heat and serve while hot. Optionally, garnish with the saved green onion tops.

Lentil and Veggie Stew

Ingredients

1 cup dried green or brown lentils, washed

1 tablespoon of olive oil.

One onion, chopped

3 minced garlic cloves and 2 peeled and chopped carrots.

2 celery stalks, chopped

One medium sweet potato, peeled and chopped

1 cup of chopped butternut squash.

4 cups low-sodium vegetable broth

1 teaspoon dried thyme.

1 teaspoon of dried oregano.

1/2 teaspoon of ground cumin

1/4 teaspoon of ground coriander.

Add salt and black pepper to taste.

2 cups chopped kale or spinach.

1 tablespoon of lemon juice.

Preparation

In a large saucepan or Dutch oven, heat the olive oil over medium heat. Sauté the onion for 3-4 minutes, until transparent.

Sauté the garlic for a further minute, until fragrant.

Combine the carrots, celery, sweet potato, and butternut squash. Cook the veggies for 5-7 minutes, stirring regularly, until they begin to soften.

Combine the rinsed lentils, vegetable broth, thyme, oregano, cumin, coriander, salt, and pepper. Heat the mixture to a boil.

Once boiling, decrease the heat to low, cover, and cook for 20-25 minutes, or until the lentils and veggies have softened.

Mix in the chopped kale or spinach and lemon juice. Cook for a further 2-3 minutes, until the greens have wilted.

Taste and adjust the seasoning as required. Serve hot.

Preparation Time

Total prep time is around 40 minutes.

Turkey Chili

Ingredients

2 tablespoons of garlic-infused olive oil.

1/2 cup chopped leek leaves (dark green only)

1 pound lean ground turkey (93 percent lean)

2 tablespoons tomato paste.

2 cups of low FODMAP chicken broth.

2 cups peeled and diced sweet potatoes (about two medium sweet potatoes)

2 medium tomatoes, cored and diced (about 2 cups).

2 tablespoons of low FODMAP taco seasoning.

1 teaspoon ground cinnamon.

1 (15-ounce) can of lentils, drained and rinsed

Add salt and pepper to taste.

Preparation

Heat the garlic-infused olive oil in a Dutch oven or soup pot over medium heat. Sauté the chopped leek leaves for 2-3 minutes, until they are brilliant green, aromatic, and tender.

Cook the ground turkey, breaking it into crumbles, until nearly thoroughly browned. Stir in the tomato paste and simmer for another minute.

Pour in the low FODMAP chicken stock, then add the diced sweet potatoes, tomatoes, low FODMAP taco seasoning, and ground cinnamon. Stir to mix.

Bring the mixture to a boil, then lower to medium-low, cover, and cook for 12-15 minutes, or until the sweet potatoes are soft.

Stir in the drained and rinsed lentils and simmer until the chili is cooked through.

Season with salt and pepper to taste.

Serve warm, topped with chopped green onion tops (green portions only), grated cheddar cheese, or crumbled corn tortilla chips.

Quinoa Salad with Grilled Chicken

Ingredients

500g quinoa

Two fresh (or frozen) chicken breasts

Two carrots.

1 Cucumber

1 red onion.

Cold-pressed olive oil, to taste.

Salt & pepper to taste.

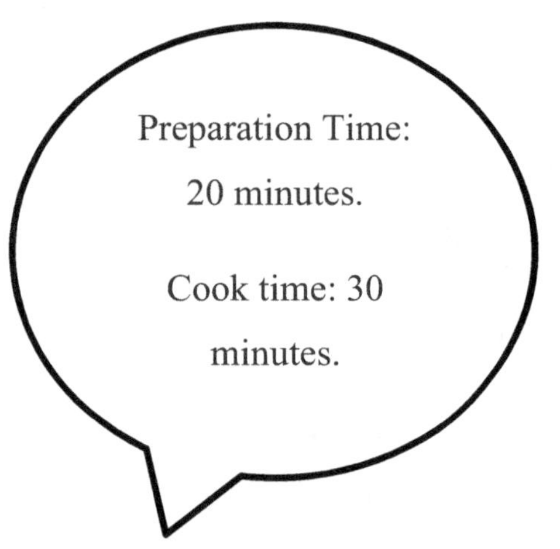

Preparation

To cook the quinoa, first rinse it in cold water.

Cook the quinoa according to package directions and put aside to cool.

Prepare the chicken.

In a frying pan, heat a little amount of cold-pressed olive oil over medium heat.

Cook the chicken breasts until golden brown and thoroughly cooked (6-7 minutes per side).

Let the chicken cool before slicing it into strips.

Chop the vegetables:

Peel the carrots and chop them into thin pieces.

Dice the cucumber into tiny pieces.

Cut the red onion in half or thin slices.

In a large dish or plate, add chilled quinoa, sliced chicken, carrot strips, chopped cucumber, and red onion.

Drizzle with olive oil, then season with salt and pepper to taste.

To serve, carefully toss together all the ingredients.

Lentil Soup with Whole Wheat Bread

Ingredients For Soup

1 tablespoon of olive oil.

1 onion, chopped

Chop 2 carrots

2 celery stalks (optional if acceptable).

2 minced garlic cloves

1 cup rinsed brown lentils

4 cups of low-sodium vegetable broth.

1 can (14.5 ounces) chopped tomatoes, fire-roasted (verify low histamine brand).

1 teaspoon dried thyme.

1/2 teaspoon dried rosemary.

Add salt and pepper to taste.

Ingredients for Whole Wheat Bread (Optional)

3 cups whole wheat flour

1 1/2 teaspoons active dry yeast

1 1/2 teaspoons salt

1 1/2 tablespoons olive oil

1 1/2 cups warm water (105°F/40°C).

Preparation

Soup:

In a large saucepan, heat the olive oil over medium heat. Cook for about 5 minutes, until the onion, carrots, and celery (if using) have softened.

Stir in the garlic and simmer for another minute.

Combine the lentils, vegetable broth, diced tomatoes, thyme, and rosemary. Bring to a boil, then decrease the heat, cover, and simmer for 30-40 minutes, or until the lentils are cooked.

Season with salt and pepper to taste.

Whole Wheat Bread (Optional)

In a large basin, combine the flour, yeast, and salt.

Combine the olive oil and warm water, and stir until a shaggy dough forms.

Turn the dough out onto a lightly floured surface and knead for 5-7 minutes, until smooth and elastic.

location the dough in an oiled basin, cover with plastic wrap, and allow to rise in a warm location for 1 hour, or until doubled in size.

Preheat the oven to 400° F (200° C). Grease the loaf pan.

Shape the dough into a loaf and place in the preheated pan.

Bake for 30–35 minutes, or until golden brown.

Cool on a wire rack before slicing.

Ingredients

4 fish fillets (about 5 ounces each)

1 pound Brussels sprouts, trimmed and halved (or quartered if bigger)

2 tablespoons olive oil.

1 tablespoon of chopped fresh rosemary (or 1/2 teaspoon dry)

1/2 teaspoon of garlic powder.

1/4 teaspoon ground thyme.

Add salt and freshly ground black pepper to taste.

Preparation

Preheat the oven to 400° F (200° C). Lightly oil a baking sheet.

In a large bowl, combine the Brussels sprouts, olive oil, rosemary, garlic powder, thyme, salt, and pepper. Spread the Brussels sprouts evenly on the prepared baking sheet.

Arrange the fish fillets on top of the Brussels sprouts.

Bake for 15-20 minutes, or until the cod flakes easily with a fork and the Brussels sprouts are soft and crunchy.

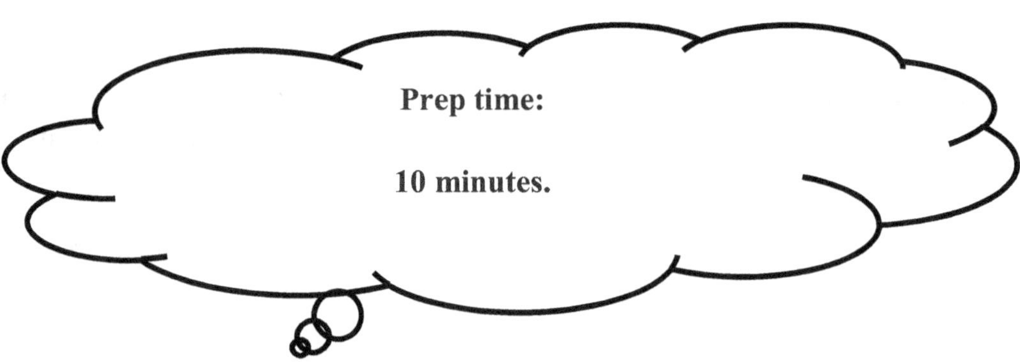

Chicken Stir-Fry with Brown Rice

Ingredients

1 tablespoon avocado oil.

1 pound boneless and skinless chicken breasts, thinly sliced

1 cup of broccoli florets.

1 cup chopped red bell peppers

1 cup of sliced zucchini.

1/2 cup chopped mushrooms (optional)

1/2 cup chopped green beans (optional)

2 garlic cloves, minced (if garlic is not accepted, substitute garlic powder).

1 tablespoon low-sodium tamari or coconut aminos.

1 tablespoon rice vinegar.

1 teaspoon ground ginger.

½ teaspoon turmeric

1/4 cup chopped fresh cilantro (optional)

2 cups of cooked brown rice.

Preparation

Cook brown rice according to the package instructions. While the rice cooks, prepare the veggies by cleaning and cutting them. Cut the chicken breasts into thin strips.

Heat the avocado oil in a large pan or wok over medium-high heat. Cook the chicken for 5-7 minutes, or until browned and cooked through. Remove the chicken from the pan and put it aside.

Place the broccoli florets, red bell pepper, zucchini, and any other veggies you're using in the pan. Cook for 3–5 minutes, or until tender-crisp.

Combine the garlic (or garlic powder), tamari, rice vinegar, ginger, and turmeric. Cook for another minute, allowing the flavors to combine.

Return the cooked chicken to the pan and toss to cover with the sauce.

Serve the stir-fry over cooked brown rice, topped with chopped fresh cilantro if preferred.

Shrimp Scampi with Zucchini Noodles

Ingredients

2 tablespoons olive oil.

3 garlic cloves, minced

1/4 teaspoon of red pepper flakes (optional)

1 pound big shrimp, peeled and deveined, tails on or off (deveined is essential for reduced histamine)

salt and freshly ground black pepper.

1/2 cup low-sodium chicken broth.

1/4 cup of dry white wine (optional; substitute extra broth if avoiding)

Juice from 1 lemon

2 zucchini spiralized into noodles (or use a julienne peeler for thin strips).

1/4 cup chopped fresh parsley.

Grated Parmesan cheese for serving (optional).

Preparation

Prep (10 minutes): Wash and spiralize the zucchini, or cut into thin strips using a julienne peeler. Set aside. Mince the garlic and cut the parsley.

Cook for 15 minutes: In a large skillet, heat olive oil over medium heat. Cook for 30 seconds, stirring in the garlic and red pepper flakes (if using), until aromatic.

Add the shrimp and season with salt and pepper. Sauté for 3–4 minutes, or until pink and cooked through. Remove the shrimp from the pan and put aside.

Scrape up any browned parts in the pan before adding the chicken broth and white wine. Bring to a boil and cook for 2-3 minutes, or until the liquid has reduced significantly.

Cook the zucchini noodles for 1-2 minutes, until tender-crisp.

Stir in the lemon juice and parsley.

Return the shrimp to the pan and toss to coat with sauce. Heat for another minute.

Serve immediately over zucchini noodles and sprinkle with grated Parmesan cheese (optional).

Salmon with Roasted Asparagus and Quinoa

Ingredients

2 salmon fillets (approx. 6 oz each)

1 bunch asparagus, trimmed

1 cup washed quinoa

1/2 cup water or low-histamine vegetable broth.

1 tablespoon of olive oil.

1/2 lemon juiced (optional)

1/2 teaspoon dried thyme.

Add salt and pepper to taste.

Preparation

Preheat the oven to 400° F (200° C). Lightly oil a baking sheet.

Pat the salmon fillets dry with paper towels. Season each side with salt, pepper, and dry thyme.

Toss asparagus with olive oil, salt, and pepper. Spread them on one half of the baking sheet.

Put the salmon fillets on the opposite half of the baking sheet.

(Optional) Drizzle the fish with a little lemon juice.

Bake for 15-20 minutes, or until the salmon is fully cooked (flaky when checked with a fork) and the asparagus is tender and crisp.

While the salmon and asparagus roast, prepare the quinoa according to package directions, using water or vegetable broth.

Once cooked, fluff the quinoa with a fork before serving with the salmon and roasted asparagus.

Prep time: 10 minutes.

Cooking Time: 20-25 minutes.

Lemon Garlic Roasted Chicken with Vegetables

Ingredients

1 entire chicken (about 3-4 pounds), fresh

2 tablespoons olive oil.

One lemon, split in half.

4 garlic cloves, peeled

1 teaspoon dried thyme.

1/2 teaspoon of sea salt.

1/4 teaspoon of black pepper.

2 cups of low-histamine veggies (such as broccoli florets, carrots, diced zucchini, or peeled and chopped butternut squash).

Prep time: 15 minutes.

Cook time: 1 to 1.5 hours.

Preparation

Preheat the oven to 375°F (190° C).

Rinse the chicken cavity thoroughly and dry it with paper towels.

In a small mixing bowl, add olive oil, lemon juice from half a lemon, thyme, salt, and pepper.

Rub the herb mixture all over the chicken, even beneath the skin (be careful).

Fill the cavity with the remaining lemon halves and garlic cloves.

Truss the chicken legs with kitchen twine (optional). This enables the chicken to cook evenly. There are video tutorials available online for trussing a bird.

Toss your choice veggies in a roasting pan with olive oil and salt.

Place the chicken, breast side up, on a bed of veggies in the roasting pan.

Roast for 1–1.5 hours, or until the thickest portion of the thigh reaches 165°F (74°C). Baste the chicken with pan drippings on occasion to add flavor and moisture.

Once done, take the chicken out of the oven and let it rest for 10 minutes before carving.

Quinoa Sweet Potato Bowl

Ingredients

1 tablespoon of olive oil.

1/2 white onion, chopped

Optional: 1 minced garlic clove.

2 medium sweet potatoes

2 diced carrots

1 diced zucchini

1 cup rinsed quinoa

1 (13.5 oz) can of coconut milk.

½ teaspoon dried thyme.

½ teaspoon dried basil.

½ teaspoon dried rosemary.

One teaspoon apple cider vinegar (or white distilled vinegar)

Pinch of salt.

A pinch of black pepper (optional).

Fresh parsley, chopped (to garnish)

Preparation

In a big saucepan or Dutch oven, bring the olive oil to a medium heat. Cook the chopped onion (and garlic, if using) for 2-3 minutes, or until softened.

Place the chopped sweet potatoes, carrots, and zucchini in the saucepan. Stir thoroughly and simmer for another 3 minutes.

Add the rinsed quinoa and toss to combine. Cook for a further minute.

Pour in the coconut milk and add just enough water to cover the contents. Bring to a boil, then decrease heat and simmer for 15 minutes, or until the quinoa is fully cooked and fluffy.

Stir in the dried thyme, basil, and rosemary. Add the apple cider vinegar and season with salt and black pepper to taste.

Pour the mixture into serving dishes and top with fresh parsley.

Prep time: 10 minutes.

Cook time: 25 minutes.

Ingredients

To make pesto

combine ½ cup of tightly packed fresh coriander leaves (cilantro).

1/2 cup pepitas (pumpkin seeds).

1/4 cup extra virgin olive oil.

1-2 cloves garlic, depending on your desire.

1 tablespoon of apple cider vinegar (optional).

Pink Himalayan salt (to taste)

Pasta:

Amount depends on your appetite (plan on 2-3 ounces per person).

Select a gluten-free option if necessary.

Preparation

Preparation (5 minutes): Wash and dry the coriander leaves. In a dry skillet over medium heat, toast the pumpkin seeds until aromatic, being careful not to burn. This step is optional, but it provides a lovely depth of flavor.

Pesto (5 minutes): In a food processor, mix all pesto ingredients and pulse until thoroughly incorporated, scraping down the sides as required. You may change the consistency by using more or less olive oil. Instead of blending continually, pulse the pesto to make it chunkier.

Cook Pasta: While the pesto is cooking, cook your preferred pasta according to package directions.

Assemble (2 minutes). Drain the cooked pasta, reserving a small amount of pasta water. Toss the pasta with the pesto, adding a splash of leftover pasta water as required to get the desired sauce consistency. Season with more salt to taste.

Fresh Fava Bean Hummus

Ingredients

2 cups fresh fava beans, shelled

1/4 cup tahini (make sure it's low in histamine)

2 tablespoons extra virgin olive oil

2 tablespoons lemon juice (optional, according on your tolerance)

1 clove garlic (optional, according on your tolerance)

Salt to taste.

Garnish with fresh herbs, such as parsley or cilantro.

> Preparation Time
>
> Total time: around 20 minutes, including boiling and chilling the fava beans.

Preparation

To prepare the fava beans, bring a saucepan of water to a boil. Cook the fava beans for about 3-5 minutes, till soft.

Drain the beans and place in a dish of cold water to chill. Once cold, remove the outer skins.

Blend the ingredients:

In a food processor, mix peeled fava beans, tahini, olive oil, lemon juice (if using), and garlic.

Blend until smooth. If the mixture is too thick, add a tablespoon of water at a time until you get the appropriate consistency.

Season with salt to taste.

Serve:

Transfer the hummus to a serving dish. Drizzle with a little extra virgin olive oil and sprinkle with fresh herbs.

Serve alongside fresh veggies, low-histamine crackers, or as a spread.

Ingredients	**Preparation**

Ingredients

1 pound cut and quartered radishes

1/4 cup of unsweetened almond milk.

2 garlic cloves, minced

1 tablespoon of olive oil.

Add salt and pepper to taste.

Preparation time: 10 minutes.

Cook time: 20 minutes.

Preparation

Prepare the radishes by trimming the ends and quartering them lengthwise.

To cook the radish quarters, cover them with water in a medium saucepan.

Bring the water to a boil over high heat, then lower to medium-low and cook for 15-20 minutes, or until the radishes are tender when pricked with a fork.

To drain and mash, place cooked radishes in a colander.

In a medium basin, mash the radishes with a potato masher or fork until they reach the appropriate consistency.

Stir in unsweetened almond milk and minced garlic until well blended.

Season and serve the mashed radish with salt and pepper to taste.

Drizzle with olive oil and serve warm.

Roasted Spaghetti Squash Boats

Ingredients

1 medium spaghetti squash (about 2 pounds)

1 tablespoon of olive oil.

¼ teaspoon sea salt

¼ teaspoon garlic powder.

¼ teaspoon dried oregano.

¼ teaspoon dry Italian seasoning.

1/2 cup mozzarella cheese (optional)

Optional sauces include pesto, roasted red pepper sauce, and low-histamine tomato sauce.

Prep time: 10 minutes.

Cooking Time: 40-45 minutes.

Preparation

Preheat the oven to 400°F (205° C).

Cut the spaghetti squash in half lengthwise with a sharp knife. Remove the seeds and any stringy parts with a spoon and discard.

Drizzle olive oil into each clean squash half and massage it very well.

Season each half evenly with salt, garlic powder, dried oregano, and Italian seasoning.

Place the squash halves, cut side up, on a baking sheet lined with parchment paper.

Roast for 40–45 minutes, or until the squash is soft and easily punctured with a fork.

Prepare your filling while the squash roasts (following low histamine recommendations). This may be sautéed ground chicken or turkey with mushrooms and spinach, or roasted chickpeas with bell peppers and zucchini.

After the squash has cooked, take it from the oven and fill each half with your preferred filling.

If desired, top with mozzarella cheese or another low-histamine cheese substitute.

Broil for 2-3 minutes, or until the cheese is melted and gently browned.

Serve immediately and enjoy!

Butternut Squash and Sweet Potato Soup

Ingredients

1 medium butternut squash (about 2 pounds), peeled, seeded, and diced.

To prepare, peel and cube three large sweet potatoes (about 1.5 lbs) and dice one large onion (approximately 1.5 cups).

4 garlic cloves, minced

5 cups veggie broth.

1 (13.5 oz) can of unsweetened coconut milk (full-fat recommended).

2 tablespoons of avocado oil.

1 ½ tablespoons salt (or to taste).

2 tsp dried rosemary.

One teaspoon of ground ginger (or two tablespoons of raw ginger)

1 teaspoon of sweet paprika (optional).

Garnishing with fresh thyme or sage is optional.

Preparation

In a large saucepan, heat the avocado oil over medium heat. Add the onions and simmer for 5 minutes, or until softened.

Add the garlic and simmer for another minute, stirring regularly.

Mix in the cubed butternut squash, sweet potato, vegetable broth, coconut milk, salt, rosemary, ginger, and paprika (if using). Bring to a boil, then lower to a simmer for 30–35 minutes, or until the veggies are cooked.

Once the veggies have been cooked, use an immersion blender or move the soup to a blender in stages and puree until smooth and creamy. You can change the consistency by adding extra broth if necessary.

Taste and adjust spices as necessary.

Serve hot, topped with fresh thyme or sage (optional).

Prep time: 15 minutes.

Cooking time: 40 minutes

Ginger Sweet Potato Carrot Soup

Ingredients

1 tablespoon of olive oil.

One medium yellow onion, chopped

2 garlic cloves, minced

1 tablespoon fresh ginger, grated

1 teaspoon of dried sage.

1 medium sweet potato, peeled and diced

Three carrots, peeled and sliced

4 cups of low-histamine vegetable broth.

Add salt and black pepper to taste.

Fresh herbs (optional for garnish): thyme, parsley, and chives.

Preparation

(5 min) In a large saucepan, heat the olive oil over medium heat. Sauté the chopped onion until translucent and softened, about 5 minutes.

** (2 min)** Put the minced garlic, grated ginger, and dried sage into the saucepan. Sauté for a further 2 minutes, stirring often to avoid scorching.

** (5 min)** Add the diced sweet potatoes and sliced carrots to the saucepan. Stir to coat the veggies in the onion, garlic, and ginger mixture. Cook for approximately 5 minutes, until the veggies begin to soften around the edges.

** (15 min)** Pour in the low-histamine veggie broth. Bring to a boil, then decrease the heat and simmer for 15 minutes, or until the veggies are soft.

** (5 min)** Once heated, either use an immersion blender or transfer the soup to a blender and puree until smooth. Season with salt and black pepper to taste.

** (optional)** Serve hot, topped with fresh herbs such as thyme, parsley, or chives (if permitted).

Crispy Zucchini Fries

Ingredients

2 medium zucchinis

2 tablespoons olive oil.

1/2 teaspoon of garlic powder.

1/2 teaspoon of sea salt.

1/3 cup tapioca starch.

Add freshly ground black pepper to taste.

Preparation

Preheat the oven to 425°F (220°C), and line a baking sheet with parchment paper.

Wash and dry the zucchinis. Cut them into thick matchsticks that are ½ inch broad and 3-4 inches long. Leave the skins on for added nutrition.

In a large mixing basin, toss the zucchini fries with olive oil until evenly coated.

Season the zucchini with garlic powder, salt, and black pepper. Toss to coat.

Toss in the tapioca starch to cover the zucchini fries evenly. Tapioca starch is an excellent alternative for breadcrumbs in a low-histamine recipe, resulting in a crunchy texture.

Spread the coated zucchini fries in a single layer on the prepared baking sheet, ensuring that they do not touch. This will allow them to crisp up evenly.

Bake for 20-25 minutes, or until the fries are golden brown and crispy. Be sure to turn the fries halfway through cooking to ensure equal browning.

Serve hot with your preferred dipping sauce, such as marinara, yogurt-based ranch dressing, or a splash of lemon juice.

SMOOTHIES

Blueberry Coconut Smoothie

Ingredients

1 cup of frozen blueberries.

1 cup of unsweetened canned coconut milk.

1/2 cup fresh spinach or kale.

¼ cup chopped banana (optional; see remark).

Add ½ cup water or more to reach desired consistency.

Ice cubes (Optional)

Stevia or monk fruit sweetener, to taste.

Bananas can be rich in histamine, so avoid them if you're rigorously following a low-histamine diet. You can test them in little quantities later to determine if they create any responses.

Preparation

Combine all items in a blender.

Blend until smooth and creamy, then add more water or ice cubes to get your preferred consistency.

Taste and adjust the sweetness with stevia or monk fruit sweetener.

Pour in a glass and enjoy!

Prep time:

5 minutes.

Ingredients

1 ripe pear with core removed

1 cup of packed fresh spinach or arugula.

½ inch fresh ginger, peeled

1 cup of unsweetened plant-based milk (almond, coconut, hemp, etc.

Ice cubes (Optional)

Instructions

(Prepare for 2 minutes) Wash and cut the pears and ginger.

(Blend for 3 minutes). Combine all ingredients in a blender and puree until smooth. If used, add ice cubes to get a thicker consistency.

Enjoy!

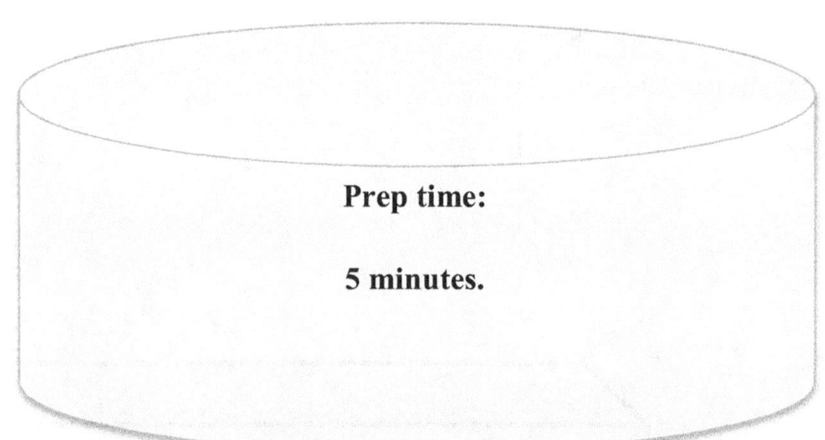

Apple Pie Smoothie

Ingredients

1 delicious apple (about 4.6 ounces)

One dried date.

1/2 cup frozen cauliflower florets.

2 tablespoons rolled oats.

1 tablespoon of macadamia nut butter.

1/2 teaspoon ground cinnamon (optional)

1-2 g fresh ginger (about ½ tsp)

1 cup of your favorite plant-based milk, such as almond or coconut.

1 tablespoon of collagen peptides (optional).

Preparation

Wash and cut the apples into bits.

Combine all items in a blender.

Blend until smooth and creamy, adding additional plant-based milk as required to get the desired consistency.

Enjoy right now!

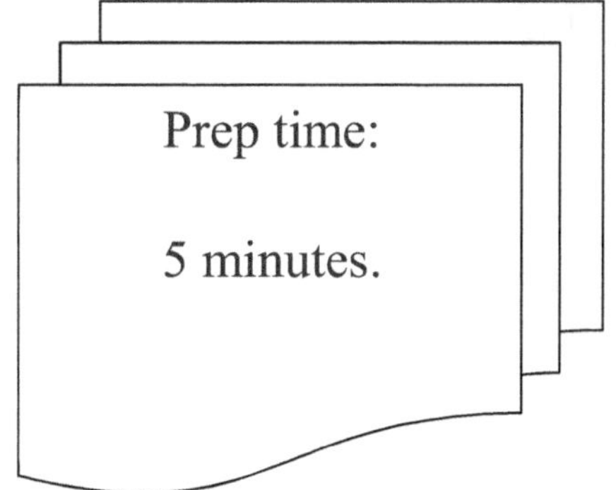

Blackberry Chard Smoothie

Ingredients

100 g blackberries, frozen or fresh.

1 small nectarine (about 150 g)

45 g cauliflower florets (frozen, or softly steamed and chilled)

30 g rainbow chard leaves, cut

1–2 tsp macadamia nut butter (or other low-histamine nut butter)

200 cc of your preferred plant-based milk (histamine-friendly choices include rice milk, coconut milk, or macadamia milk)

Optional add-ins:

1–2 tsp collagen peptides (for additional protein)

1 tsp acacia fiber (to increase thickness and intestinal health)

Preparation

Wash and cut the nectarines, removing the pit.

Wash and coarsely slice the rainbow chard leaves.

Blend all of the ingredients until smooth.

Taste and adjust the sweetness or thickness as needed with additional milk or a little water.

Enjoy right now!

Pomegranate Juice Smoothie

Ingredients

1 cup blueberries, fresh or frozen.

1/2 banana, peeled and frozen.

1/2 cup pomegranate seeds.

1 cup unsweetened low-histamine yogurt (coconut yogurt or kefir are good options)

1 cup plant-based milk (histamine-free alternatives include rice, almond, or oat milk)

Optional:

1 tablespoon ground flaxseed (added fiber)

A pinch of ground ginger (for anti-inflammatory benefits)

Preparation

Combine all items in a blender.

Blend until smooth and creamy, adding additional plant-based milk as required to get the desired consistency.

Enjoy right now!

Mango Spinach Smoothie

<table>
<tr><td>

<u>Ingredients</u>

1 ½ cups fresh baby spinach.

1 cup of frozen mango chunks.

¼ cup plain or vanilla low-fat Greek yogurt (optional; see note).

1 cup unsweetened vanilla almond milk (or low-histamine milk)

1/2 teaspoon ground ginger (optional)

Honey or maple syrup (to taste, optional).

</td><td>

Preparation

Combine all items in a blender.

Blend on low speed at first, using a tamper if needed, until well blended.

Increase the speed to medium-high, and mix until extremely smooth.

If desired, sweeten with honey or maple syrup.

Pour in a glass and enjoy!

</td></tr>
</table>

Please keep in mind that Greek yogurt may contain a lot of histamine. If you are particularly sensitive, you can eliminate it or substitute a low-histamine yogurt, such as coconut yogurt.

Prep time:

5 minutes.

Pear and Basil Smoothie

<table>
<tr><td>

Ingredients

One ripe pear, cored and diced

1 cup of fresh basil leaves.

1 cup of oat milk (or other low-histamine milk of your choice).

1 tablespoon of chia seeds.

1 teaspoon fresh ginger, grated

One teaspoon of pure monk fruit powder (optional for sweetness)

A pinch of salt.

</td><td>

Preparation

Pour the pear, basil leaves, oat milk, chia seeds, ginger, monk fruit powder, and salt into a blender.

Blend on high speed for 1-2 minutes, or until smooth.

Pour into a glass and drink immediately.

</td></tr>
</table>

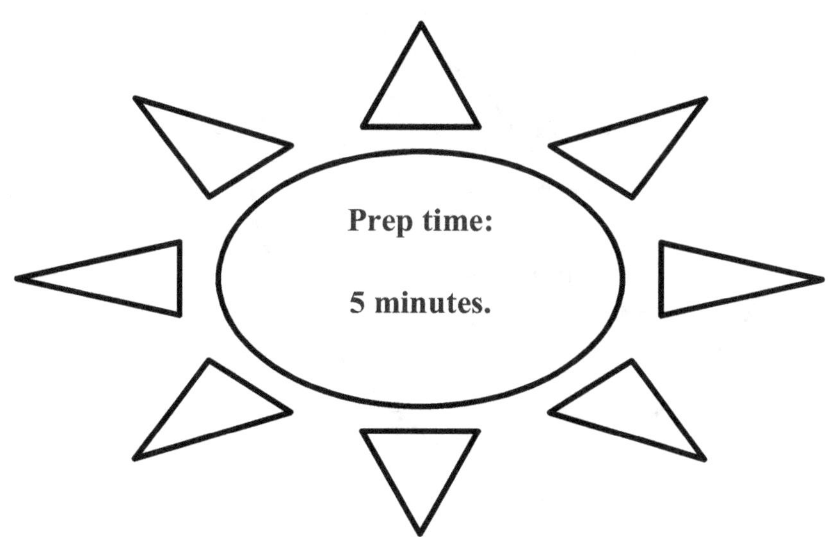

Cucumber Mint Smoothie

<table>
<tr><td>

<u>Ingredients</u>

One medium cucumber, peeled and cut

1/2 cup of fresh mint leaves.

One green apple, cored and cut

1/2 avocado.

1 cup coconut water (or any low-histamine drink of your choice)

1 tablespoon of chia seeds.

1 teaspoon of fresh lemon juice.

A pinch of salt.

</td><td>

Preparation

Place the cucumber, mint leaves, green apple, avocado, coconut water, chia seeds, lemon juice, and salt in a blender.

Blend on high speed for 1-2 minutes, or until smooth.

Pour into a glass and drink immediately.

</td></tr>
</table>

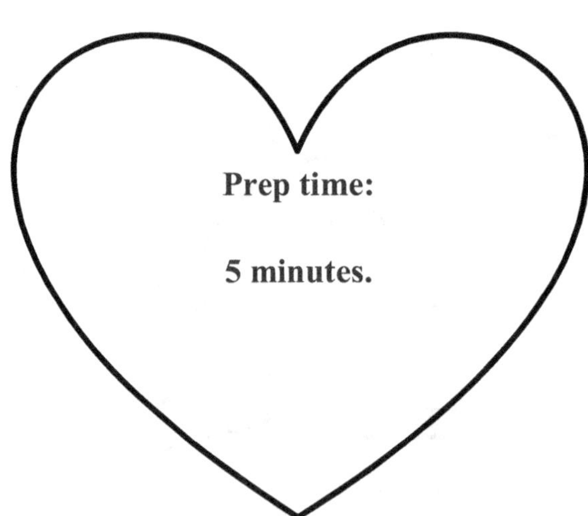

Strawberry Banana Smoothie

Ingredients

1 cup fresh, hulled strawberries

One ripe banana.

1 cup coconut milk (or other low-histamine milk you want)

1 tablespoon of chia seeds.

1 teaspoon of pure vanilla essence.

A pinch of salt.

Preparation

Combine the strawberries, banana, coconut milk, chia seeds, vanilla essence, and salt in a blender.

Blend on high speed for 1-2 minutes, or until smooth.

Pour into a glass and drink immediately.

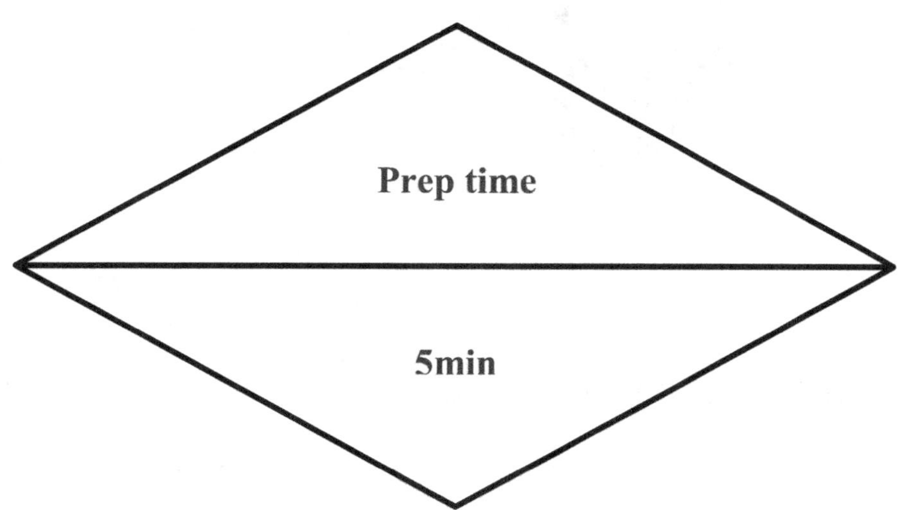

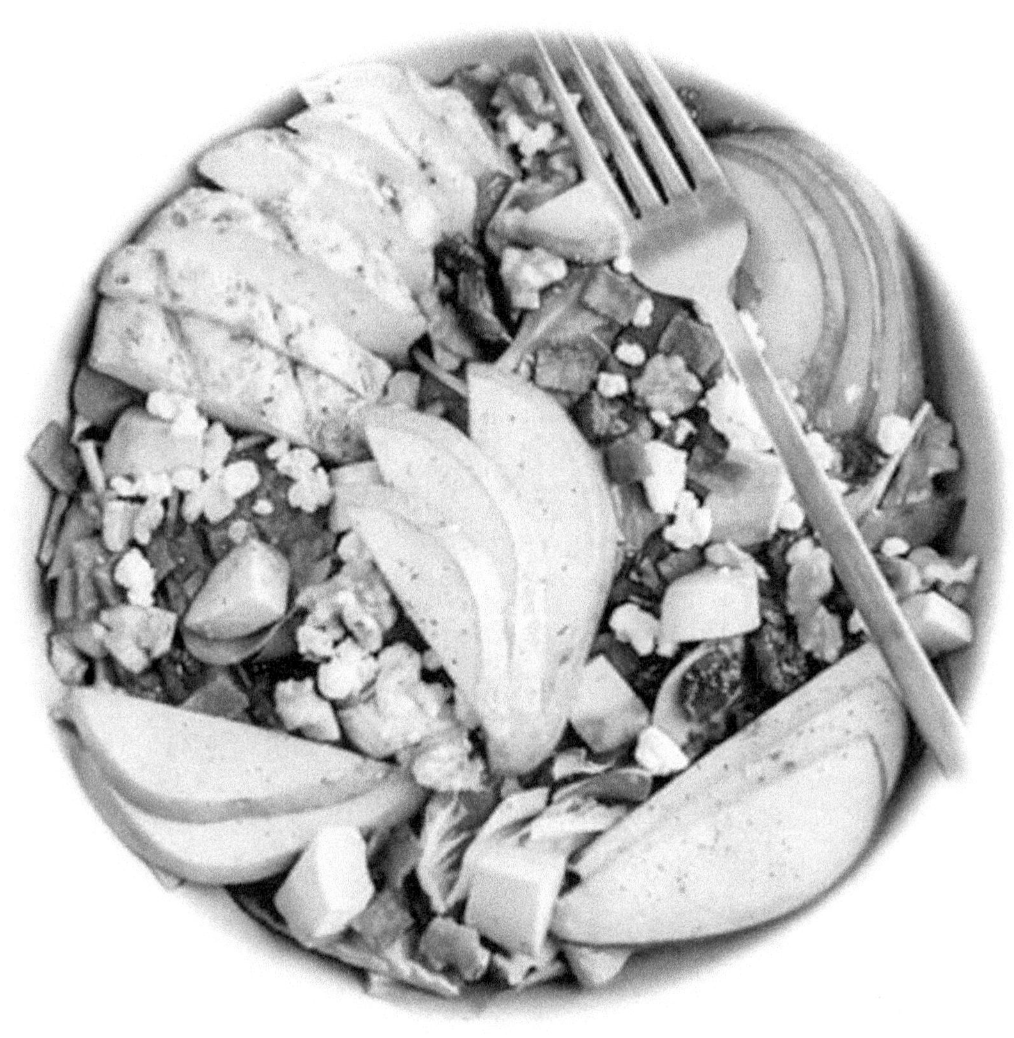

THANKS FOR YOUR PURCHASE, HOPE YOU ENJOYING SOME OF THIS RECIPES.

COULD YOU PLEASE TAKE A FEW SECONDS TO LEAVE A HONEST FEEDBACK ON THIS BOOK

CONCLUSION

Congratulations! You have reached the end of your gastronomic journey into the realm of histamine intolerance. We've looked into the science of histamine, investigated its effects on health, and provided you with important ways for managing it properly. More significantly, we've demonstrated that a life full of wonderful food and bright health is entirely attainable, even with histamine sensitivity.

This book has more than simply low-histamine recipes. It's a road map to empowerment, providing you with the information and resources you need to navigate your own unique journey. Here are some of the benefits you get by purchasing this book:

Empowerment through Knowledge: Understanding the facts underlying histamine intolerance enables you to make educated dietary and lifestyle decisions. You'll go from feeling dissatisfied and powerless to empowered and in command of your health.

Farewell Frustrating Symptoms: By recognizing triggers and following the procedures provided in this book, you can greatly lessen the frequency and severity of histamine-related symptoms. Imagine waking up feeling rejuvenated, eating without discomfort, and recuperating your energy for things you like.

A World Of Delicious Possibilities: Low-histamine does not have to be tasteless! This book is packed with delectable, easy-to-follow recipes that accommodate to a wide range of dietary needs. Rediscover the joy of cooking and appreciate delectable meals that feed your body and satisfy your palate.

Histamine intolerance may have been a hardship, but it also provided a chance for good development. By accepting this journey and applying the ideas suggested in this book, you may live a healthier, more vibrant life. You'll learn to listen to your body, select meals that make you feel well, and rediscover the pleasure of cooking and eating. Let this book serve as your culinary compass, bringing you to a world of delicious independence from histamine mayhem.

So put on your chef hat, take a fresh item, and set off on this gastronomic journey of self-discovery. Remember that with education, good food, and a positive attitude, you can live a life in which histamine intolerance does not restrict you; rather, it enables you to become a healthier, happier you!